Physiological Principles in Medicine

General Editors

Professor M. Hobsley
Department of Surgical Studies, The Middlesex Hospital and
The Middlesex Hospital Medical School, London

Professor K.B. Saunders
Department of Medicine, St George's Hospital and St George's Hospital
Medical School, London

Dr J.T. Fitzsimons
Physiological Laboratory, Cambridge

Disorders of the Kidney and Urinary Tract

Physiological Principles in Medicine

Books are published in linked pairs – the preclinical volume linked to its clinical counterpart as follows:

Endocrine Physiology by Richard N. Hardy
Clinical Endocrinology by Peter Daggett

Digestive System Physiology by Paul A. Sanford
Disorders of the Digestive System by Michael Hobsley

Respiratory Physiology by John Widdicombe and Andrew Davies
Respiratory Disorders by Ian R. Cameron and Nigel T. Bateman

Neurophysiology by R.H.S. Carpenter

Reproduction and the Fetus by Alan L.R. Findlay
Gynaecology, Obstetrics and the Neonate by S.J. Steele

Body Fluid and Kidney Physiology by S.B. Hladky and T.J. Rink
Disorders of the Kidney and Urinary Tract by F.D. Thompson and C.R.J. Woodhouse

Disorders of the Kidney and Urinary Tract

F.D. Thompson
Consultant Nephrologist, St Peters Group of Hospitals, London and Harefield Hospital; Dean, Institute of Urology, London, UK

and

C.R.J. Woodhouse
Senior Lecturer, The Academic Unit, Institute of Urology, London, UK; Consultant Urologist, St George's and St James's Hospitals, London, UK and The Royal Marsden Hospital, London, UK

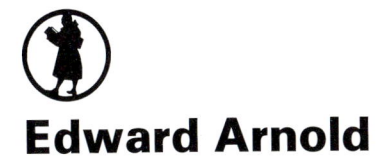

Edward Arnold

© F.D. Thompson and C.R.J. Woodhouse 1987

First published in Great Britain 1987 by
Edward Arnold (Publishers) Ltd, 41 Bedford Square, London WC1B 3DQ

Edward Arnold (Australia) Pty Ltd, 80 Waverley Road, Caulfield East,
    Victoria 3145, Australia

Edward Arnold, 3 East Read Street, Baltimore, Maryland 21202, U.S.A.

British Library Cataloguing in Publication Data

Thompson, F.D.
   Disorders of the kidney and urinary tract.
   — (Physiological principles in medicine)
   1. Genito-urinary organs — Diseases
   I. Title   II. Woodhouse, C.R.J.
   III. Series
   616.6   RC871

ISBN 0-7131-4412-2

All rights reserved. No part of this publication may be reproduced, stored in a retrieval system, or transmitted in any form or by any means, electronic, photocopying, recording, or otherwise, without the prior permission of Edward Arnold (Publishers) Ltd.

Whilst the advice and information in this book is believed to be true and accurate at the date of going to press, neither the authors nor the publisher can accept any legal responsibility or liability for any errors or omissions that may be made.

Text set in 10/11pt Baskerville Compugraphic
by Colset Private Ltd, Singapore
Printed and bound by Butler & Tanner Ltd, Frome and London.

In Memory
Dr R.N. Hardy

General preface to series

Student textbooks of medicine seek to present the subject of human diseases and their treatment in a manner that is not only informative, but interesting and readily assimilable. It is important, in a field where knowledge advances rapidly, that principles are emphasized rather than details, so that what is contained in the book remains valid for as long as possible.

These considerations favour an approach which concentrates on each disease as a disturbance of normal structure and function. Rational therapy follows logically from a knowledge of the disturbance, and it is in this field where some of the most rapid advances in Medicine have occurred.

A disturbance of normal structure without any disturbance of function may not be important to the patient except for cosmetic or psychological reasons. Therefore, it is disturbances in function that should be stressed. Preclinical students should aim at a comprehensive understanding of physiological principles so that when they arrive on the wards they will be able to appreciate the significance of disordered function in disease. Clinical students must be presented with descriptions of disease which stress the disturbances in normal physiological functions that are responsible for the symptoms and signs which they find in their patients. All students must be made aware of the growing points in physiology which, even though not immediately applicable to the practice of Medicine, will almost certainly become so during the course of their professional lives.

In this Series, the major physiological systems are each covered by a pair of books, one preclinical and the other clinical, in which the authors have attempted to meet the requirements discussed above. A particular feature is the provision of numerous cross-references between the two members of a pair of books to facilitate the blending of basic science and clinical expertise that is the goal of this Series. This coordination, which is initiated at the planning stage and continuous throughout the writing of each pair of books, is achieved by frequent discussions between the preclinical and clinical authors concerned and between them and the editors of the Series.

MH
KBS
JTF

Preface

Dramatic advances in technology since the Second World War, and especially in the last 20 years, have opened up new fields of investigation in all medical disciplines; patients with diseases of the urogenital tract have been particularly fortunate. Nuclear imaging, computerized axial tomography (CAT scanning) and intra-luminal pressure measurements (urodynamics) have made diagnosis far more accurate and improved our knowledge of physiology. Treatment too has been improved and become much less unpleasant: new membranes for haemodialysis, shock wave destruction of stones and efficient optics for endoscopic surgery are obvious examples.

In spite of such modern wonders, our basic approach to patients has not changed. Good medicine is still based on the best traditions of history, examination and judicious use of investigations. Diagnosis and treatment may be much improved but modern science must never be a substitute for a good 'doctor and patient relationship'.

Clinical medicine still requires a sound knowledge of normal physiology. The changes produced by disease, the pathophysiology, can be then understood. Exact mechanisms may still elude the research worker, but it is from his discoveries that the student can appreciate the symptoms and signs of disease.

The companion volume to this text (Hladky and Rink *Body Fluid and Kidney Physiology*, Edward Arnold, London) has outlined the essentials of renal physiology. In this book the pathophysiology and its application to clinical problems is described.

All common diseases of the urogenital system have been covered, with a pathophysiological emphasis. It is not intended as a comprehensive volume, but one that will guide the student with his first nephrological and urological patients. In particular the references only form a guide to the literature that is available for detailed reading.

It is our intention that the text can be read easily and, with the appetite whetted, more knowledge will be sought in this fascinating and rewarding area of clinical medicine.

1986   FDT
CRJW

Contents

General preface to the series	vii
Preface	viii
Contents of *Body Fluid and Kidney Physiology* by S.B. Hladky and T.J. Rink	xii
1 Patient assessment	**1**
Patient history	1
Physical examination	3
Macroscopic urine analysis	4
Microscopic analysis of urine sediment	5
Glomerular filtration rate	7
Renal blood flow	7
Tubular function	8
2 Imaging in urology	**10**
Anatomical investigations	10
Physiological investigations	14
3 Acute renal failure	**20**
Pathophysiology	20
Investigations	22
Clinical management	25
The recovery phase	30
4 Chronic renal failure	**31**
Aetiology	31
Clinical assessment	32
Management	34
Substitution therapy	39
5 Dialysis	**40**
Haemodialysis	40
Haemofiltration	43
Peritoneal dialysis	44

x   Contents

6 Transplantation	**48**
Immunology	48
Clinical signs of rejection damage	49
Measures to prevent rejection damage	50
Surgical procedure	52
Postoperative management	52
7 Proteinuria and glomerulonephritis	**57**
Histological classification of glomerulonephritis	58
Immunology	61
Clinical presentation	62
Common forms of glomerulonephritis	63
Nephrotic syndrome	68
8 Systemic hypertension	**71**
Aetiology	72
Renal artery stenosis	73
Hypertension associated with renal disease apart from renal artery stenosis	76
Non-renal causes of hypertension	76
Assessment of end-organ damage	77
9 Infections of the urinary tract	**82**
Cystitis	82
Symptomless bacteriuria	85
Management of specific problems of cystitis	85
Prostatitis	86
Epididymo-orchitis	87
Renal infections	88
Genitourinary tuberculosis	91
10 Obstruction	**95**
Signs and symptoms	95
Kidney obstruction	98
Ureteric obstruction	101
Bladder obstruction	102
Prostate enlargement	103
Obstructive lesions in children	104
Medical management	104
11 Disorders of bladder function	**106**
Normal bladder function	106
Obstructions to outflow	108
Neuropathic lesions	114
Incontinence	117
Urinary diversion	120

12 Congenital anomalies	**123**
Renal anomalies	123
Renal pelvic and ureteric anomalies	124
Bladder anomalies	130
Urethral anomalies	131
The testes	132
13 Male infertility and impotence	**136**
Infertility	136
Impotence	140
14 Tubular disorders	**151**
Specific tubular defects	151
Acquired tubular defects	155
15 Renal disease in general medicine	**158**
Diabetes mellitus	158
Vasculitis	159
Amyloid deposition	162
Multiple myeloma	163
Gout	164
Sarcoid lesions	165
Pregnancy	165
16 Pharmacology	**167**
Principles	167
Nephrotoxicity	169
17 Cancer of the genitourinary tract	**171**
Haematuria	171
Cancer of the kidney	173
Cancer of the urothelium	178
Cancer of the prostate	185
Cancer of the testis	189
Cancer of the penis	193
Further reading	**194**
Index	**199**

Contents of *Body Fluid and Kidney Physiology* by S.B. Hladky and T.J. Rink

While reading this book you might find it helpful to refer to the companion volume, *Body Fluid and Kidney Physiology*. The following list of contents will enable you to look up the physiological background to the material contained in this book.

1. The body fluids
2. The relations between the body fluids and the mechanisms for the transfer of substances between them
3. Basic structure of the kidneys and mechanisms of urine production
4. Methods for studying renal function
5. Glomerular filtration
6. The transport functions of the proximal tubule
7. The transport functions of the distal tubule and the collecting system
8. The production of dilute or concentrated urine
9. Hormonal and metabolic functions of the kidney
10. The regulation of the body fluids by the kidneys
11. Nitrogenous wastes and foreign substances
12. Potassium, calcium, magnesium, phosphate, and sulphate
13. Osmoregulation
14. Control of extracellular fluid volume, blood volume, and the intake and excretion of sodium
15. The role of the kidneys in the regulation of blood pressure
16. Regulation of pH
17. The role of the kidneys in pH regulation

1

Patient assessment

A patient with a renal problem may remain free of symptoms until the disease is well advanced. The patient may then seek medical advice, complaining of malaise, weight loss and anorexia; and at that point the glomerular filtration rate (GFR) may be reduced to approximately one-third of normal, accompanied by a rise of blood urea. This 'silent' loss of function is common, and with such a late presentation little can be achieved with conservative treatment.

Routine medical examinations for employment and insurance purposes often uncover renal problems when hypertension and proteinuria are detected, and in this group early detection affords the best chance that treatment will prevent further damage.

There are, however, certain features which can be gleaned from accurate history taking and examination which point towards renal pathology. This process should not be overlooked or replaced by modern techniques of investigation, as it not only produces valuable information but also promotes a rapport with the patient – essential if long-term care is to be effective. It is valuable for the student to have a framework for history taking and examination, and such a framework relevant to the renal patient will now be described.

Patient history

Alterations in the pattern of micturition may provide early clues. Urinary frequency if associated with dysuria suggests infection. The volumes voided on each occasion are important: small volumes suggest an irritable, unstable bladder, while large volumes in keeping with polyuria may be associated with chronic renal failure and both forms of diabetes, mellitus and insipidus. The passage of urine immediately after the bladder has been emptied may be due to refilling of the bladder from a diverticulum or from refluxed urine draining down from a dilated upper urinary tract. Nocturia may only reflect late-night drinking, but it may also be secondary to impaired concentrating ability seen in chronic renal failure and congestive cardiac failure.

Disorders of bladder outflow produce difficulty in initiating micturition, a poor stream and post-micturition dribbling. Incontinence is an obvious abnormality which may simply reflect retention of urine with overflow or a more complex pathology (see Chapter 11).

The presence of a significant amount of protein may cause freshly voided urine to appear frothy and an abnormal discoloration may be reported by the patient. The common causes are listed in Table 1.1. Spectroscopic confirmation by the laboratory will be required.

If pain is a presenting feature then the type, location and radiation often provide diagnostic clues. Loin pain, which can be severe and may radiate anteriorly, suggests obstruction at the pelviureteric junction and such a pain may be made worse following a high fluid intake. Unilateral loin pain, when accompanied by fever and rigors, points towards upper tract infection, while loin pain made worse by micturition suggests major vesicoureteric reflux. The renal parenchyma itself is not rich in pain fibres, and it is stretching of the renal capsule which produces these symptoms. Ureteric colic is severe and often radiates anteriorly towards the pubis, down to the testicles and often down the anterior aspects of the thighs. Its colicky nature is caused by waves of ureteric peristalsis which are trying to propel small stones, blood clot or debris down to the bladder, and this pain is so severe that once experienced it is never forgotten. Bladder tumours and inflammation may cause suprapubic discomfort, and if this is accompanied by spasm the patient experiences urgent and frequent desires to micturate, which may in itself be painful – strangury. Urethral disease may be associated with pain, and often if infection is the cause a urethral discharge results. Prostatic infection causes deep-seated perineal and rectal pain.

Oedema is a common presenting feature. Ankle and lower limb oedema may be due to mechanical, venous or lymphatic obstruction or cardiac failure, and the hypoproteinaemia of the nephrotic syndrome may produce severe pitting oedema of the whole leg. Facial oedema is more common in children. In addition to the visual impression of oedema, the gain in weight is an absolute and accurate guide to the efficacy of treatment. Approximately 3–6 litres of fluid may be retained before obvious oedema is noticed, but a significant weight gain is more easily detected. Early pulmonary oedema produces the typically irritating non-productive cough before obvious dyspnoea becomes apparent. In the renal patient, fluid overload associated with sodium and water retention as well as simple hypertensive left ventricular failure are common aetiological factors. Ascites may also be present in these patients.

A past medical history may illuminate the current problem. Childhood fevers suggest reflux pyelonephritis, while a previous history of hypertension,

Table 1.1 Discoloration of urine

Red:	Haematuria, free haemo- or myoglobin, drugs (e.g. rifampicin and phenothiazines)
Purple:	Porphyria
Brick red:	Urate (often as a sediment only)
Brown:	Bile, haematuria
Green:	Methylene blue and amitriptyline
Black:	Melanin, falciparum malaria
White:	Phosphate (sediment only), pus, chyle

diabetes, tuberculosis or gout, for example, may suggest that the kidney has been involved by these general medical conditions. As will be discussed in detail later, a history of self-administered or prescribed drugs is important as analgesics, antibiotics etc. may all be nephrotoxic, and vitamin D found in many proprietary medicines may be a factor in stone formation. An enquiry into the health of the immediate family may suggest hereditary disease, such as polycystic disease, hereditary nephritis, hyperoxaluria and renal acidosis. Occupational hazards (e.g. the use of organic solvents and hydrocarbons) may produce tubular damage and predispose to bladder cancer.

Physical examination

As each system is examined in detail, the following signs may be of specific interest.

General

Anaemia, bruising, hyperpigmentation and excoriation of the skin and pale, white lines across the nails (Mee's lines) are often features of chronic renal failure.

Cardiovascular system

Peripheral oedema, hypertension which may only be apparent on standing or taking exercise, and postural hypotension are not solely confined to those patients with a peripheral neuropathy; they may reflect a low circulating volume which is due to a sodium-losing condition.

Evidence of right or left ventricular failure is important. The patient with a low cardiac output may have renal impairment directly as a result of poor cardiac function – the energy for glomerular filtration being generated by the left ventricle. Sub-acute bacterial endocarditis may be associated with embolic renal disease or a glomerulonephritic process. A pericardial rub present in severe uraemia is of interest, but of greater importance are the features of cardiac tamponade.

Respiratory system

A nasal discharge and necrotic septum are seen in Wegener's granulomatosis and deep, sighing respiration (Kussmaul) is seen in severe acidosis. Dyspnoea at rest is often associated with the auscultatory findings of pulmonary oedema as mentioned above. Pleural effusions can be detected clinically, while haemoptyses associated with pulmonary haemorrhage are obvious and are associated with Goodpasture's syndrome.

Abdomen

The kidneys move on respiration and it is only the lower pole of the right kidney in normal subjects that is readily palpable. Enlarged kidneys are often palpable. The enlargement may be due to obstruction, cystic disease or tumour, for example.

The liver may also be enlarged owing to cystic disease, amyloid or secondary tumour.

Shifting dullness associated with ascites is obvious if the collection of fluid is large, and a large bladder is often easy to palpate and percuss. In women this must be distinguished from uterine or ovarian pathology, and re-examination after bladder catheterization is often of value. The prostatic size can often be assessed by rectal examination provided that the bladder is empty, and exquisite tenderness is present in cases of prostatitis. Urine culture after prostatic massage may produce the causative organism.

Central nervous system

Nerve deafness suggests hereditary nephritis, and the fundal changes associated with hypertension are self-explanatory.

During an eye examination, evidence of corneal calcification associated with the abnormal calcium homeostasis of chronic renal failure may be apparent.

Macroscopic urine analysis

Accurate ward or out-patient testing provides information that should not be spurned. The tests should, if possible, be carried out by the physician in charge of the patient as this will ensure that they are performed with interest and accuracy.

In health, osmolality is in the range 50–1200 mosmol/kg depending on the state of hydration. If a hydrometer is used this range is represented by values between 1.001 and 1.040. A reasonably large volume is required, and the use of a refractometer provides more accurate information from a small volume of urine. The most accurate value will come from depression of the freezing point, which is a laboratory technique. Glucose, mannitol, iodinated contrast media and heavy proteinuria will produce falsely elevated readings.

pH

This can be measured easily using indicator papers or a pH electrode. Values of 5 confirm normal acidification, while values greater than 7 suggest alkali therapy, infection or renal tubular acidosis.

Glucose

A dipstick procedure is used which depends on a colour reaction produced by peroxidase. Cross-reaction with other urinary constituents may give falsely low readings. The enzymes are specific and eliminate the false positive results which bedevil the use of Benedict's solution. Ketones can also be detected by a similar technique.

Protein

Dipsticks are available which react specifically with albumin and which give a rough quantitative value. Under-estimation occurs in an alkaline urine. Tubular protein, globulins and light chain fragments produced in myeloma do not react, but these can be detected by precipitating with salicylic acid. However, accurate qualitative and quantitative information will be produced by the laboratory using specific antisera and electrophoretic techniques. The molecular size is important and an index of selectivity will provide prognostic information. Further details will be found in Chapter 7.

Haemoglobin

Haemoglobin can be detected by a dipstick procedure which is extremely sensitive. Red cell morphology is important and is seen when freshly voided urine is examined under the microscope.

Microscopic examination of urine sediment

Valuable information can be gained from microscopy of freshly passed urine. A more formal assessment is obtained when the sediment is resuspended from a centrifuged deposit (15 ml of urine for 3 minutes at 5000 rev/min). The laboratory can take this investigation further by the use of electron microscopy which may detect amyloid fibrils, and special cytological techniques will define accurately the cell types. However, much information can be gained by the physician personally, and this information, which costs little, should be obtained in a side room of the ward or in the out-patient department.

Red cells

These are seen in many conditions – stones, tumour, infection, etc. Those which have forced their way through an abnormal glomerulus are misshapen and can be detected by phase contrast microscopy. Those produced by lower tract bleeding have a normal morphology. Red cells per high power field can be quantified.

Leucocytes

Many polymorphs can be seen and may suggest general inflammation, as seen in pyogenic infection and transplant rejection.

Tubular epithelial cells

These are normally present but are increased in numbers in conditions with predominant parenchymal damage, such as acute renal failure and interstitial nephritis.

Bladder squames

These, too, are normally present but are increased and abnormal in cases of neoplasia. Specialist cytological techniques are extremely valuable.

Vaginal squames

These are a normal contaminant.

Proteinacious casts

Usually composed of Tamm–Horsfall protein, these are casts of the tubular and collecting duct lumens. Large, broad casts are seen in cases of obstruction and renal failure. Smaller casts may have any of the above cellular elements adhering to their surface. Again the number of casts can be quantified and this will give a rough guide as to severity.

Fat droplets

These may be present in the nephrotic syndrome and in cases of heavy proteinuria. They may be ingested by macrophages and are often easily detectable by phase contrast.

Bacteria, yeasts, Trichomonas, etc.

These may be seen in heavy infections.

Crystals

Crystals of characteristic shapes are often present in patients with renal calculi, and a higher yield of crystals can be obtained in the laboratory when the urine is concentrated by evaporation. Calcium, phosphate, triple phosphates and ammonium urate crystals are commonly seen in an alkaline urine, while an acid urine produces crystals of oxalate, urate, uric acid and cystine.

A combination of various deposits is also of value in diagnosis. With acute glomerulonephritis, red cells and white cells associated with numerous tubular and red cell casts are seen in large numbers, while with chronic renal failure the cellular content is often low and large hyaline casts predominate. Large numbers of polymorphs and organisms suggest infection, and here a careful collection of a mid-stream urine for culture is obviously important. In order to rule out possible contamination during the collection of specimens in difficult cases, fine-needle aspiration of a full bladder suprapubically is often of great value. Acid-fast bacilli are often more easily detected if the early-morning concentrated urine is sent for culture by specific techniques.

Glomerular filtration rate

Formal assessment of renal function is clearly important, both in the initial assessment of the patient and to follow the effect of treatment. While the majority of tests relate to the measurement of the glomerular filtration rate, assessment of tubular function is of equal importance, especially as a diagnostic aid.

The clearance of a substance which is freely filtered at the glomerulus and ignored by the tubules will provide a measure of the glomerular filtration rate. A timed urine collection of a 12–24 hour sample plus a venous measurement will allow the standard formula $(U \times V)/P$ to be used, where U is the urine concentration, V is the volume per unit time and P is the plasma concentration (Hladky and Rink, pp. 4–5 and 37–8).

Endogenous creatinine derived from muscle is the standard compound that is measured. In cases of heavy proteinuria, tubular secretion may occur, and in renal failure various other accumulated compounds may interfere with the chemical measure; but creatinine clearance is still – despite these disadvantages – the routine technique.

Infusion of inulin and vitamin B_{12} have been used, but a steady plasma concentration has to be reached and this can only be achieved over a limited time. Hence the urine collections are shorter and the measurements less accurate.

Reliability is lost if the urine collection is not accurate; and since it is often surprisingly difficult to obtain carefully timed collections from patients, isotopic techniques using the rate of disappearance from the bloodstream are becoming more widely accepted. A substance such as EDTA (ethylene-ditetra-acetic acid) labelled with Cr^{51} is freely filtered at a glomerular level and is not reabsorbed or secreted by the tubules. A known amount is injected cleanly intravenously, and blood samples taken at 0, 20 and 40 minutes. The volume of distribution and

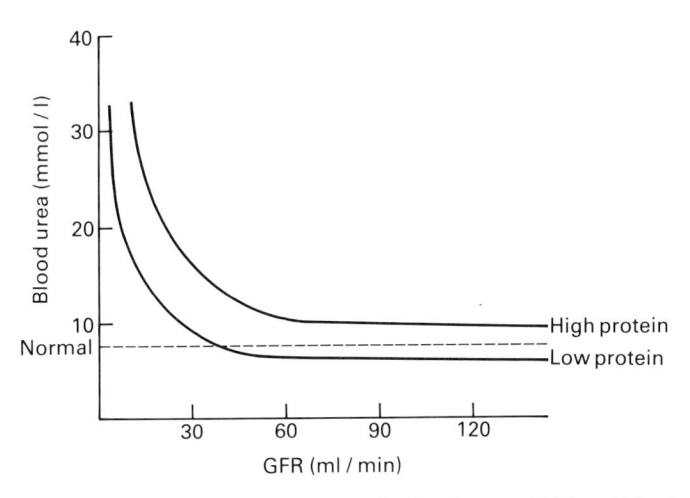

Fig. 1.1 Relationship between glomerular filtration rate (GFR) and blood urea concentration (in mmol/l), according to whether the subject is on a high or low protein diet.

the glomerular filtration rate can be calculated, since after the first 10 minutes the disappearance from the bloodstream relates directly to the glomerular filtration rate. This technique does away with the problems of urine collection, but it has the disadvantage that injection extravasation produces gross inaccuracies, and the presence of oedema renders the technique inaccurate. These clearance techniques are required as the plasma concentrations of urea and creatinine do not have a linear relationship with the glomerular filtration rate (Fig. 1.1).

In addition the blood urea is influenced by the state of hydration, dietary protein intake, liver function and drugs such as tetracycline and steroids. Serial creatinine values are more reliable in following changes in GFR as long as the muscle mass does not change significantly. However, as with urea concentration, there is not a major increase until two-thirds of the glomerular filtration rate is lost, and then further small reductions will produce a disproportionate rise in the plasma concentration. Some clinicians find the reciprocal plot of the plasma creatinine a more useful guide to the change in the glomerular filtration rate.

Renal blood flow

Using the Fick principle it is possible to equate the clearance of PAH to the effective renal plasma flow (Hladky and Rink, pp. 38–9). This technique is not used in clinical practice. In the course of renal scintigraphy using diethylene triamine pentacetic acid (DTPA) Cr^{51} it is possible not only to define the renal tract anatomy but also to produce an index of renal perfusion, along with estimates of the overall GFR and individual renal function. This renal perfusion index is not an absolute value for renal blood flow; but nevertheless it is extremely useful in monitoring changes in blood flow in the transplanted kidney, and it is of value in the diagnosis of renal artery stenosis.

Tubular function

Urine concentration

Specific gravity and urine osmolality measurements have been mentioned. As a formal test of concentrating ability the urine osmolality should rise to at least 600 mosmol/kg following a 12-hour fast. If this figure is not achieved, it is possible to assess tubular function following the injection of Pitressin or desamino D-8 arginine vasopressin (DDAVP).

Urine dilution

The response to an oral fluid load as a test of urine dilution can be physically dangerous. As urine dilution also depends on normal adrenal function, this non-specific test is rarely performed.

Urine acidification

If a random pH of 5 or below is reached, then a major fault in hydrogen ion secretion is unlikely. If there is any doubt the response to oral ammonium chloride (0.1 g/kg) is measured. The pH should fall to below 5.2. (Hladky and Rink, pp. 203, 206, 211-12.)

Urine electrophoresis

This can be performed to isolate abnormal amino acids such as cystine, leucine and valine. Calculation of the maximum absorptive capacity of the renal tubules (T_M) is rarely performed (Hladky and Rink, pp. 39-41), but in abnormalities of urine acidification the T_M bicarbonate can be measured. Similarly the T_M glucose may be diagnostically valuable in cases of glycosuria not caused by diabetes mellitus.

2

Imaging in urology

The technology of 'imaging' has developed so rapidly in the last ten years that traditional ideas of investigation in most specialties have been radically changed. In urology the intravenous urogram has passed from its long-held premier position to being one of several equals.

In any programme of investigation a basic sub-division can be made into specific diagnostic tests and assessments of general condition: this chapter deals only with the former. Although it is useful to 'pigeon-hole' patients according to their presenting problems and thus, mentally, trigger off a particular series of tests, it is equally essential to stop the series when the relevant questions have been answered. In ordinary clinical practice there is no need to continue the investigations to satisfy a predetermined and often arbitrary programme.

Urological imaging techniques can be broadly divided into 'anatomical' and 'physiological'. The abundance of techniques that are available makes it even more important than usual to decide what questions are to be answered before planning the tests.

The following sections will consider imaging techniques specifically related to the genitourinary tract.

Anatomical investigations

Plain abdominal X-ray

The information obtained from a test is often inversely proportional to its 'sophistication'. The plain abdominal radiograph certainly obeys this rule of thumb. The patient is placed supine on the X-ray table and one or more films are taken to include the abdomen from the top of the left kidney to the bottom of the urethra. This area is too large in about 50 per cent of adults to fit on a single film.

In looking at these films, as with any other X-ray, a scheme should always be followed that ensures that all the available information is picked up. The clinician's natural excitement at finding, for example, a staghorn calculus must not mean that an osteolytic metastasis in the lumbar spine is missed.

Aside from the non-urological lesions, the plain films are principally of value in conditions of altered mineral deposition. In practice this almost always means calcification, which may be seen in almost any urological lesion but is associated particularly with chronic infection, local ischaemia and stones.

The intravenous urogram (IVU)

Preparation

It used to be routine for patients to take a laxative, to be starved and dehydrated for 12 hours before an IVU. Without this preparation the small doses of contrast that were used did not show up the kidneys through the overlying bowel shadows. However, the use of high doses of iodine containing contrast media has made preparation of the patient less important. Some departments still give a laxative the night before, but dehydration is seldom employed and is definitely contraindicated in patients with renal failure, diabetes or multiple myeloma.

Physiology of contrast media

Radio-opaque contrast medium is given intravenously. The radio-opaque component is based on iodine, and is carried in a solution usually based on sodium. For the majority of patients there is little to choose between the commercially available media, most of which are based on sodium diatrizoate. With normal renal function at least 300 mg/kg of iodine is needed (600 mg in renal failure), a volume of 70–100 ml. The solutions are hyperosmolar and should be avoided in patients with heart failure. In infants, especially when they are very ill, the osmolar load is dangerous; and as the IVU gives little useful information in this group, it has rightly disappeared from neonatal practice.

The contrast media are glomerular-filtered and there is negligible tubular handling. The amount filtered is proportional to the plasma level of contrast. The concentration by the kidney is due to tubular reabsorption of water.

Complications

Virtually all patients feel sensations of warmth and nausea immediately after contrast injection. A few patients have a 'reaction' which may be extremely severe or even fatal. The reaction begins within a few minutes and consists of vasodilatation, urticaria, bronchospasm, hypotension and, in severe cases, cardiac arrest. The mechanism is unknown; it does not appear to be a true allergy as it may occur with the first exposure to contrast and not with subsequent exposures.

Treatment should be given immediately with intravenous antihistamine and hydrocortisone. If necessary the patient should be intubated and ventilated.

If there is a mild reaction, subsequent IVUs should be covered with prophylactic antihistamines and steroids. If the reaction is severe, the examination should not be repeated (even though the reaction might not occur again).

Information provided

The IVU remains the mainstay of urological investigation, but it provides much 'anatomical' and little 'physiological' information. It is an excellent guide to further investigation. There are three phases to the IVU:

Nephrogram. When the contrast is being filtered the kidneys are shown and their shape is seen. A delayed nephrogram suggests diminished blood supply and a prolonged nephrogram indicates obstruction or acute tubular necrosis.

Pyelogram. When the contrast fills the calyces, renal pelvis and ureters their shape and size are seen. It must be most definitely understood that dilatation of the collecting system does not always mean that it is obstructed.

Bladder phase. The contrast takes a variable time to reach the bladder. If the bladder has been incompletely emptied the contrast will not mix freely with the bladder urine, but, being denser, sinks to the bottom giving a false impression of bladder size and shape. Otherwise the bladder shape is seen, but it must be remembered that it is a large 3-dimensional organ being seen on a 2-dimensional film. The outline can only be properly judged when the bladder is reasonably full.

A further bladder film is taken after voiding, as tumours are often more clearly seen. The fact that fewer than 70 per cent of IVUs on patients with invasive bladder cancer show any abnormality is an indicator of how poorly the bladder is seen on an IVU.

The micturating cystourethrogram (MCU)

If the bladder is filled with a water-soluble contrast through a urethral or suprapubic catheter, better views of the bladder are obtained. In cases of suspected cancer no information is provided that will not be obtained by cystoscopy, and MCU is seldom performed to get anatomical information about the bladder. However, it is very good at picking up vesicoureteric reflux and for looking at the anatomy of the urethra. If possible, the act of voiding should be watched on the image intensifier.

The residual urine seen on the post-micturition film either after MCU or IVU is a poor guide to the true residual for several reasons. The bladder is usually incompletely filled during an IVU and filled too fast with cold contrast for an MCU, before the patient is asked to void. During an IVU the patient is sent to void quickly in a fairly public lavatory – often with a radiographer of the opposite sex waiting outside the door. During an MCU the patient must void on the table in front of the camera. It is hardly surprising that a poor performance is produced. If the bladder is emptied it shows that it can be done, but if a residual remains it proves little. A massive residual is usually significant, but this could probably have been seen on a good plain film.

The urethrogram

A jelly contrast injected retrogradely down the urethra gives an excellent definition of the distal end of a urethral stricture. Because inadequate contrast may get past the stricture, its true length may be difficult to judge. To get an accurate picture of the whole stricture it is best to combine a urethrogram with an MCU.

In females it is seldom necessary to obtain an X-ray of the urethra. The rare condition of urethral diverticulum can usually be seen on MCU.

The vasogram

In a few cases of infertility it is necessary to confirm the patency of the vas (see Chapter 13). The vas is exposed in the scrotum and injected with contrast through a fine needle.

The ureterogram

Improvement in the technique of IVU has led to better visualization of the ureter, so that a ureterogram is indicated less and less often. If a ureter is draining a kidney with reasonable function it is usually possible to fill the ureter by IVU. If this fails the ureter can be filled with contrast either antegradely by percutaneous puncture of the renal pelvis, or retrogradely by catheterization of the ureteric orifice via a cystoscope. Both procedures are hazardous, especially in unskilled hands, and should only be undertaken when other alternatives have been tried.

Antegrade ureterogram

This investigation is usually done under local anaesthesia by a radiologist. If the kidney is large (as from an obstruction) it is fairly easy to locate it with a needle without any special aids. For a smaller target it is better to try to visualize the system with intravenous contrast or to puncture under ultrasound control. Once the needle is in, contrast is injected after aspiration of urine. If necessary the needle can be replaced by a plastic tube for short- or long-term drainage.

Retrograde ureterogram

This investigation has become less common in recent years. Retrograde catheterization of the ureteric orifice via a cystoscope is relatively easy under general anaesthetic, but it can be difficult under local anaesthetic. If the system is obstructed, infection can easily be introduced with dire consequences. The forceful injection that is often made through ureteric catheters may rupture the ureter or renal pelvis.

Computed tomography (CT scan)

The CT scan marries the well-established techniques of X-ray with the computer. The radiographic part of the apparatus generates a series of tomographic images focussed at serial depths through the body. The computer converts them into cross-sectional pictures of the body at predetermined intervals.

14 *Imaging in urology*

Because the pictures show all the organs of the body, giving detailed anatomical information, it is tempting to use a CT scan as the initial investigation in all cases of obscure diagnosis. This is a misuse of an invaluable but expensive tool. The principal value of CT scanning in urology is for the definition of cancers and their metastases.

Ultrasonography

Ultrasound has been widely used in medicine for only 10 years, but its use by animals for locating objects and navigating has been known for 200 years. Ultrasound waves are generated by applying an alternating current to certain crystals (quartz and tourmaline were the first to be used by Pierre Curie in the 1880s). Returning waves vibrate the crystal to generate an electric current.

For medical imaging, frequencies of between 1 and 10 megahertz (MHz) are used. Waves travel through tissue at 1.5 mm per microsecond. The waves are reflected at each interface between tissues with different mechanical properties. The intensity of the reflection is proportional to the square of the difference of the acoustic impedances of the two tissues: thus an interface between two different soft tissues is poorly defined by ultrasound, but that between a soft tissue and a fluid is very well defined. Waves of these frequencies do not penetrate bone.

The equipment for generating and displaying ultrasound waves is developing rapidly, but even now, ultrasonography has displaced conventional radiography in the investigation of many urological problems, especially in infants and children. It is painless, non-invasive and harmless. Its only real drawback is that it is difficult for anyone except the operator to interpret the images, so that the clinician has no visual evidence to back up the written report.

The main uses of ultrasonography may be deduced from the foregoing description. Renal cysts can be distinguished from tumours with 98 per cent accuracy; dilatation of the urinary tract and sites of narrowing can be identified and followed after voiding or catheterization; some stones can be found and the local spread of some prostatic and bladder cancers can be defined; and biopsy or aspiration needles can be accurately positioned under ultrasound control.

Physiological investigations

Isotope scans and renography

The handling of compounds labelled with radioactive isotopes by the urinary tract can be followed by scintigraphy counters (which produce a graph) or by gamma cameras (which produce a picture). Urinary tract transport function can be observed and renal function measured.

^{131}I-hippuran renogram

Hippuran is filtered by the glomeruli and secreted by the tubules so that its rate of uptake by the kidney gives a measure of renal perfusion and function. Its most important use, however, is in following the passage from renal parenchyma to bladder with appropriately positioned probe scintigraphy counters. In spite of many criticisms that have been laid against this technique, it is still one of the most reliable methods of identifying obstruction.

^{99m}Tc-DTPA

Diethylene triamine pentacetic acid (DTPA) is handled entirely by glomerular filtration. Sequential gamma-camera pictures after a bolus injection show, successively, renal blood flow, parenchymal uptake and glomerular filtration. A computer can quantify the uptake and provide a measure of relative function between the two kidneys. Delay in the vascular phase indicates renal artery stenosis.

Once it is in the glomerular filtrate DTPA is unaltered, and its removal from the kidney is entirely dependent on the dynamic function of calyces, pelvis, ureter and bladder. Sequential gamma-camera pictures are used to identify obstruction. The effects of obstruction can be accentuated by increasing the urine flow with a diuretic such as frusemide. A computer can measure the transit time across particular parts of the urinary tract (areas of interest) to define sites of obstruction more precisely.

^{99m}Tc-DMSA

Dimercaptosuccinate (DMSA) is retained in the renal cortex for a long time and is slowly excreted through the tubules. Gamma-camera pictures taken soon after a bolus injection give similar information to that provided by DTPA. Later pictures define areas of functioning cortex. The technique is useful in identifying and monitoring renal scars, particularly in children, and distinguishing tumours from pseudo-tumours.

Antegrade pressure studies (Whitaker test)

An agreed mathematical definition of upper tract obstruction has proved elusive. Although it would seem simple enough to measure the ability of the transport system to transmit the urine from collecting tubules to bladder, the many variables involved have given rise to dispute about the figures produced. Furthermore, the effects of obstruction on renal function have been difficult to quantify.

The comparison between renal pelvic and intravesical pressures at a flow rate of 10 ml/minute under standardized conditions is generally accepted as the 'gold standard' of upper tract obstruction. The technique is commonly called the Whitaker test, after its inventor.

The apparatus is shown diagrammatically in Fig. 2.1. A bladder catheter is used both to measure pressure and to fill and empty the bladder: upper tract obstruction may only be apparent with a full bladder. The needle is positioned in the renal pelvis under X-ray control. The pelvis is perfused at 10 ml/minute. A pressure difference between pelvis and bladder of less than 10 cm H_2O indicates no obstruction, 10–20 cm is equivocal, and over 20 cm indicates obstruction. It is essential to continue the perfusion for long enough to fill the

16 Imaging in urology

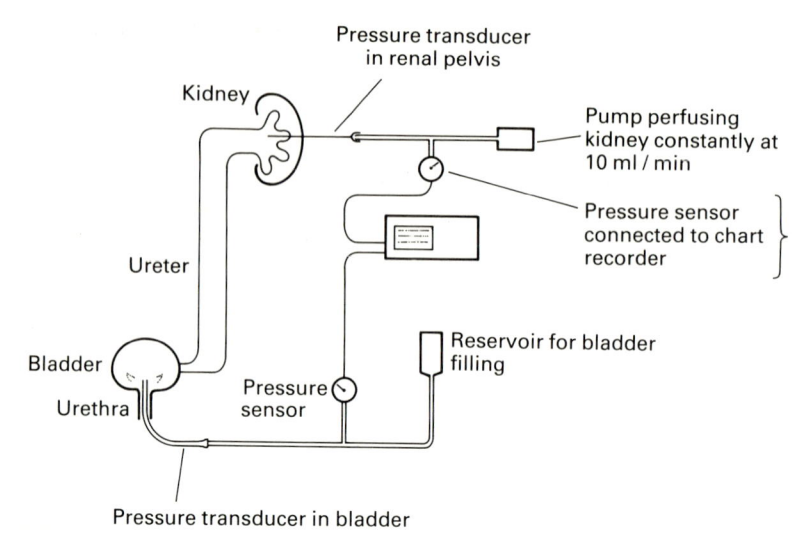

Fig. 2.1 Apparatus for renal/bladder pressure measurements (Whitaker test).

whole collecting system with saline before the pressure is measured.

The Whitaker test is invasive and requires time and patience to perform. Long-term follow-up of patients has confirmed its accuracy. A DTPA scan with Lasix (a diuretic) compares favourably, but both tests have false positives and negatives. In cases with near normal renal function and relatively acute obstruction, the scan is the investigation of choice. In more complex cases with poor renal function and chronically dilated collecting systems, only the Whitaker test will distinguish between sluggish flow and true obstruction.

Lower tract pressure studies (urodynamics)

Much of our knowledge of the physiology of the bladder and urethra has come from experimental and clinical measurements of intraluminal pressures. Added sophistication comes from simultaneous cystourethrography (the video cystometrogram) or electromyographic recordings of the sphincters and pelvic muscles.

Flow rate

In the past, much ingenuity has gone into attempts to measure the rate at which the bladder is emptied. An average flow is easy to measure, but it is the peak flow that is of importance. Commercially available flow meters have now solved the problem: voiding into a flow-sensitive receiver disguised as a lavatory is translated into a flow rate such as that in Fig. 2.2. 18 ml/second is generally taken as the lower limit of normal.

The flow rate must be considered together with the patient's symptoms and age and is not of great diagnostic value on its own. It does provide an objective

Cystometrogram

The object is to measure the pressure generated by the detrusor muscle during bladder filling and emptying and with provocations such as coughing and changing posture. The test requires two urinary catheters – one as a pressure transducer and one for bladder filling – and a rectal transducer, so that the pressure generated by the abdominal muscles can be subtracted from the total intravesical pressure to give the pressure generated by the detrusor. The test is combined with flow rate measurement. The transducers are connected to a continuous recorder that can subtract the rectal from the detrusor pressure and produce a graph of pressure against volume (Fig. 2.2).

The presence of the various catheters and the surrounding apparatus might suggest that the results would not be representative of normal bladder function. Nevertheless, the results are reproducible, are clinically relevant, and the investigation has stood the test of time.

Video cystometrogram

This test combines the cystometrogram with the micturating cystourethrogram. Simultaneous video recording of pressure and shape allows anatomical and physiological information to be correlated; in particular, sites of obstruction can be seen. The test may be further combined with electromyography to identify abnormal sphincter or pelvic muscle behaviour.

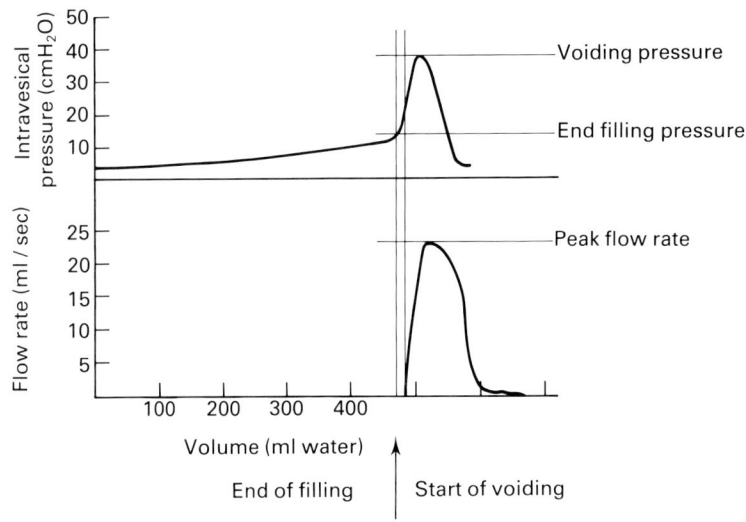

Fig. 2.2 Sample traces of intravesical pressure (with intra-abdominal pressure subtracted) and flow rate in a normal patient.

Urethral pressure profile

Knowledge of the pressure generated by the urethral sphincters at rest, and in response to rises in intravesical pressure, is useful in defining causes of incontinence. An open-ended and perfused catheter, connected to a pressure transducer, can be drawn slowly out from the bladder neck to produce a profile of urethral pressure at a given time.

Recently, very fine catheters with a series of pressure transducers along their length have become available. These allow intravesical and urethral sphincteric pressure to be measured continuously. The response to various provocations, particularly rising intravesical pressure, can be seen.

These techniques have yet to establish a place in routine urology, but they are invaluable in specialized clinics.

Nuclear magnetic resonance (NMR)

The next exciting development on the horizon is nuclear magnetic resonance. This non-invasive and, it is said, totally harmless investigation provides anatomical and biochemical information. A few machines are undergoing clinical evaluation, and it is already clear that it will be an invaluable tool in urological investigation.

Atoms with an odd atomic number have an electric charge and an intrinsic property of spin, and they thus produce a very small magnetic field. In practice, only hydrogen (atomic number 1) is present in high enough concentration in the body to produce a measurable magnetic field. At rest, the magnetic fields are randomly arranged so that they cancel each other out, and the net magnetic vector is zero. If the body is placed in a strong magnetic field most of the magnetic vectors line up parallel with the direction of that field, and the spinning protons of each atomic nucleus will spin around the axis of the magnetic field. The axis of spin can now be altered by applying a radio wave with a frequency equal to the frequency of the spin. When this happens, the spinning protons absorb energy and release it when the radio wave is switched off. This release of energy is called magnetic resonance and is measurable. The magnetic resonance is altered by the biochemical environment of the atoms and by their position in the external magnetic field.

How this complex set of physical properties is translated into visual and biochemical information of clinical relevance is beyond the scope of this text. The inevitable computer and attendant software, most of which was originally developed for CT scanning, does the work. In essence it is measuring the responses of the hydrogen nuclei to varying magnetic fields and radio frequencies.

Although the pictures generated look similar to those from a CT scanner, the NMR scanner is much more sensitive and so provides finer anatomical detail. As the direction of the magnetic field is infinitely variable, the body can be scanned in any plane. The distinction between different tissues is sufficiently marked that conventional contrast media are not needed.

Very few NMR scanners are in clinical use and so their clinical role is not fully known. Full anatomical detail of the urinary tract is better shown than with

CT-scanning. The small biochemical differences that are detectable may allow the monitoring, or even the diagnosis of, inflammatory conditions such as glomerulonephritis; certainly the distinction between renal cortex and medulla is clearly seen. Particularly good definition of the local extent of tumours throughout the genitourinary tract is available, and there is an advantage over CT-scanning in that there is no distortion by bone or surgical clips. In the future, measurement of blood and urine flow rates will introduce a new dimension of combined physiological and anatomical imaging.

3
Acute renal failure

Acute renal failure may be defined as the rapid reduction in renal function that had previously been normal. Some patients presenting to their doctor for the first time may have pre-existing renal disease and the sudden deterioration may represent the final stages of chronic renal failure. The distinction between *de novo* acute renal failure and acute upon chronic failure will become apparent as the appropriate investigations are performed.

The prognosis of acute renal failure has improved with the advent of supportive dialysis. In those cases in which the renal failure is secondary to trauma or major surgery, the overall prognosis is often poor, and to give the patient the optimum chance of survival an understanding of the underlying pathophysiology is essential. Once renal failure is established the clinical care will include careful conservative management, detailed investigation and possibly supportive measures in the form of haemo- or peritoneal dialysis. This chapter will outline the principles of patient management, having first considered the possible underlying pathophysiology.

Pathophysiology

There are many reasons why a patient may develop acute failure. The aetiological factors are classified below on an anatomical basis.

Blood vessels

The major renal vessels may be involved in a dissection of the aortic wall, and if this dissection extends into the renal arteries then blood flow may cease. Blood flow may also be impaired as the result of emboli associated with mitral stenosis, bacterial endocarditis or a mural thrombus on the surface of a myocardial infarct. Local thrombus formation may occur in cases of atherosclerosis and aneurysm. The lumina of the smaller interlobular vessels are occluded in cases of scleroderma, polyarteritis nodosa and the haemolytic uraemic syndrome.

Glomeruli

The arterioles and the capillary loops may be rapidly occluded by fibrinoid

Table 3.1 Conditions that may be associated with acute tubular dysfunction

Trauma following major surgery	Myoglobinuria
Crush injuries	Abortion
Burns	Concealed accidental haemorrhage in pregnancy
Peritonitis	
Acute pancreatitis	Hypotension associated with myocardial infarction
Mismatched blood transfusion	
Hepato-renal syndrome	

necrosis in malignant hypertension. Proliferation of the endothelial or epithelial cells in a rapidly progressive form of glomerulonephritis may occur and prevent filtration.

Tubules

The tubules may be damaged functionally and anatomically in a large number of conditions, grouped together in Table 3.1. Such damage has been known for several years as 'acute tubular necrosis'; but on examination of renal biopsies from patients with this condition, major necrosis is certainly not a prominent feature. Macroscopically the kidney is swollen and oedematous. By light microscopy the glomeruli are frequently normal but the tubules are dilated. The basement membrane is fragmented, but if any necrosis is seen it is minor and of a patchy distribution. A better descriptive name would be 'acute tubular dysfunction'.

No single concept can account for the anuria that develops. Several mechanisms may be involved. Cortical ischaemia is an important factor. In cases of hypovolaemia and hypotension the blood supply to the kidney is reduced in order to maintain cerebral and coronary blood flows. Blood is shunted away from the cortex where filtration at the glomeruli normally occurs. This has been elegantly demonstrated in the experimental animal when, during controlled haemorrhage, the development of gradual cortical ischaemia has been demonstrated radiographically. This cortical vasoconstriction is possibly mediated by sympathetic nerve stimulation and the release of catecholamines, and perpetuated by the powerful vasoconstrictor angiotensin II – a result of renal ischaemia stimulating the renin–angiotensin system. These agents cause endothelial swelling, sludging of red cells within the capillaries and interstitial oedema. In some cases intravascular coagulation produces further stasis within the renal vasculature. In extreme cases these factors combine to produce patchy necrosis of the outer cortex. This is typically found during pregnancy in cases of concealed, accidental haemorrhage, although extensive cortical necrosis has also been reported in cases associated with head injuries, burns and gastrointestinal haemorrhage. In children, however, peritonitis, profuse diarrhoea and vomiting have been known to produce severe cortical ischaemia.

Bacterial toxins released during septicaemia, and various chemical agents (Table 3.2), can cause tubular damage. However, the changes produced by toxins in ischaemia do not produce tubular necrosis as such and, as previously stated, acute tubular dysfunction is a better descriptive title. The changes

22 Acute renal failure

Table 3.2 Chemical agents known to cause direct tubular damage

Mercuric salts	Sulphonamides
Bismuth	Antibiotics
Carbon monoxide	polymixins
Carbon tetrachloride	amphotericin B
Arsenic	kanomycin
Phosphorus	cephaloridine
Ethylene glycol	gentamicin
Diethylene glycol	Contrast media for radiology
Insecticides	Some anaesthetic agents (e.g.
Barbiturates	methoxyflurane)
Salicylates	

associated with this condition that lead to oliguria are by no means clearly defined. However, it is possible that tubular damage is sufficient to allow leakage of the glomerular filtrate straight into the interstitium, producing oedema and a rise in the interstitial pressure. This pressure rise may be sufficient to compress renal vessels and ultimately prevent filtration at the glomerulus.

In cases of acute tubular dysfunction, light microscopy often shows a cellular infiltrate in the interstitium, consisting of lymphocytes, monocytes and polymorphs. A predominantly interstitial reaction is seen in cases of streptococcal and staphylococcal septicaemia, and this may in part represent an infection of the renal parenchyma itself. An eosinophilic reaction is seen in cases of drug toxicity, antibiotics in particular being incriminated. It is difficult to distinguish, however, between the effects of the septicaemia itself and those of the antibiotics that are prescribed as therapy.

Urinary tract obstruction

Upon sudden cessation of urine flow, obstruction to the urinary tract has to be excluded as a cause. This subject is dealt with fully in Chapter 10.

Investigations

A detailed history will, of course, provide valuable information. The patient who has complained of a severe sore throat some 10–14 days previously may well have a post-streptococcal glomerulonephritis, a previous history of ureteric colic may point to obstruction, while a history of septicaemia or hypotension associated with trauma and surgery supports a diagnosis of acute tubular dysfunction.

The distinction between physiological oliguria and acute tubular dysfunction

When a patient who is oliguric (i.e. passing less than 400 ml/24 hours), it is vital to decide whether this is a normal response by the kidney in order to conserve fluid, or a direct result of intrinsic renal disease. The former is a

Table 3.3 Characteristics of the urine in physiological oliguria and acute renal failure

	Physiological oliguria	Acute renal failure
Urine/plasma urea ratio	>20:1	<10:1
Urine/plasma osmolar ratio	>2:1	<1.2:1
Urine sodium concentration	<20 mmol/l	>30 mmol/l

normal physiological response by a healthy kidney and the treatment will be fluid replacement. In the latter, overhydration might already be present and further administration of fluid may be lethal.

The necessary distinction can be made easily and rapidly by the analysis of a sample of plasma and urine collected simultaneously. The major differences are set out in Table 3.3. If the urine volumes are reduced to 0.5 ml/minute in an attempt by the kidney to conserve fluid in cases of dehydration, then the urine osmolality will be high, reaching values of 500–600 mosmol/kg. When this is compared with the normal plasma osmolality, it can be seen that the urine: plasma ratio (U/P) is greater than 2:1. The concentration of urinary urea will also be high; compared with the concentrations found in plasma, a U/P ratio of greater than 20:1 can be expected. This is in direct contrast to the values obtained in a case of acute tubular dysfunction when the ability to pass a concentrated urine is lost and, despite a rising blood urea, the U/P ratio is below 10:1. The urinary sodium concentration may also be of value, as in cases of physiological oliguria the urinary concentration is low whereas in intrinsic renal failure it is set at a higher level, often around 30 mmol/litre or greater. The reasons for this latter setting are not clear.

When mannitol, dextrose or contrast medium has been given for an IVU, the urine osmolality must be interpreted with caution as these substances are freely filtered and will be responsible for an apparently high urine osmolality.

At this point mention must be made of polyuric renal failure. Not all cases of acute tubular dysfunction present with oliguria. In some cases, mainly those secondary to septicaemia, pancreatitis and burns, urine volumes in excess of 600 ml/24 hours (sometimes far greater) are produced. This urine contains little urea and creatinine, and despite these high volumes the plasma urea and creatinine continue to rise.

Urine microscopy and culture

These investigations may provide valuable information. In cases of acute glomerulonephritis, granular and red cell casts can be seen, and if polyarteritis is present 'telescoped deposit' may be noted (see Chapter 7). In inflammatory lesions large numbers of polymorphs and organisms may be seen and the latter cultured. In cases of intrarenal infection organisms are not always cultured from the urine, and so a negative culture must not be relied upon to exclude an infective aetiology.

The IVU

The carefully performed intravenous urogram (IVU) provides much valuable information (see Chapter 2). The plain film may demonstrate renal calculi, and the presence of a nephrogram excludes major vascular obstruction. The nephrogram phase, which represents contrast being concentrated within the tubules, may persist for several hours. In cases of suspected obstruction, if films are taken up to 24 hours following the injection, then the typical appearance of dilated calyces and ureter may be seen.

Radiology will allow an estimate of renal size to be made by measurement of the polar length. In adults this should approximate to the length of three and a half lumbar vertebrae; and if the kidneys are small, then this suggests the presence of pre-existing renal disease and it may be that the acute renal failure has been superimposed upon chronic renal damage. The chances of recovering adequate renal function in this situation are greatly reduced.

On occasion polycystic renal disease is demonstrated, and kidneys that have a smooth outline and are larger than normal are suggestive of renal involvement with multiple myeloma or amyloid.

These investigations should be carried out on all new cases of acute renal failure. If obstruction is suspected at this stage, further investigations are required. A diagrammatic outline of possible investigations is set out in Fig. 3.1.

Definition of possible obstruction

In cases of sudden and complete anuria, obstruction has to be excluded as a cause. A delayed IVU film may give a great deal of valuable information as to whether obstruction is present and its possible anatomical site. Chapter 10 deals in detail with obstructive uropathy; here we can note that a cystoscopy and ureterography will be required. If the obstruction is prostatic and the surgeon has succeeded in passing a catheter past any obstruction, then it can be left in situ in order to allow drainage and renal function to improve before corrective surgery.

A better alternative to retrograde ureteric examination is the antegrade pyelogram in which, under local anaesthetic and X-ray control, a needle is passed percutaneously into the dilated renal pelvis; whereupon, following the injection of contrast, the site of obstruction is often clearly defined. A catheter can be left in situ, again relieving the obstruction, allowing the clinical condition of the patient to improve prior to surgery.

The non-invasive ultrasound technique often provides useful information as to the site of obstruction as the dilated pelvis and ureter can often be delineated with this technique.

The probe renogram can demonstrate obstruction if reasonable filtration is taking place behind the obstructed lesion. The use of the gamma camera with a computer-assisted readout will provide useful information in the future since it may be possible not only to define the anatomical site of the obstruction but also to measure overall and individual kidney function.

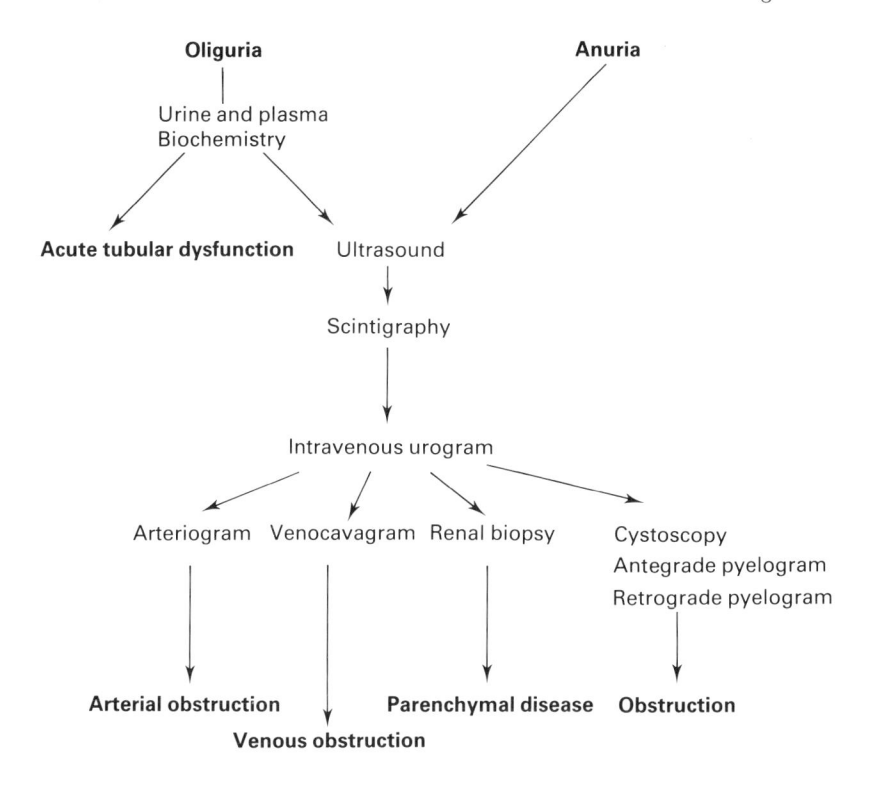

```
              Oliguria                         Anuria
                 |                              /
          Urine and plasma                    /
            Biochemistry                    /
           /     |      \                 /
          /      |       \              /
Acute tubular dysfunction   Ultrasound
                               |
                               ↓
                          Scintigraphy
                               |
                               ↓
                       Intravenous urogram
              /         /        \              \
             /         /          \              \
       Arteriogram  Venocavagram  Renal biopsy   Cystoscopy
            |           |             |          Antegrade pyelogram
            |           |             |          Retrograde pyelogram
            ↓           ↓             ↓                ↓
     Arterial obstruction     Parenchymal disease   Obstruction
              Venous obstruction
```

Fig. 3.1 Possible lines of investigation in acute renal failure.

Angiography

Impairment of the blood supply to the kidney by embolism or dissection of the renal vessels can often be detected by examination of the IVU, renogram and by gamma-camera studies. If doubt remains then angiography will be required. On occasions this is an important question; if an elderly patient is being supported by haemodialysis, there is obviously no chance of recovery if the kidney is ischaemic, and the question of long-term supportive measures will have to be carefully discussed.

Renal biopsy

When the history and earlier investigations leave uncertain the aetiology of acute renal failure, then a percutaneous renal biopsy is indicated. Acute glomerulonephritis may be present, and this will require specific treatment.

Clinical management

The management of acute tubular dysfunction from whatever cause will be considered in detail. The general principles are also applicable to cases of obstruction, malignant hypertension or glomerulonephritis, but these require in addition specific treatment regimens that will be considered elsewhere.

Diuretic challenge

In a few cases the early use of diuretics may prevent acute renal failure from becoming established. With a bladder catheter in situ, the osmotic diuretic mannitol (200 ml of a 25% solution) can be given by a rapid intravenous infusion. If this is successful, a diuresis will occur within 10-15 minutes. Care must be taken to ensure that the patient's circulation will stand the infusion of this osmotic load, and there is little to be gained by repeated infusion.

If this infusion fails then the loop diuretic frusemide may be given as an intravenous bolus injection of 40-80 mg; and if this fails the diuretic challenge may be completed by giving ethacrynic acid (50 mg i.v.). Over recent years high doses of frusemide have been given intravenously, and some success has been achieved by employing a constant i.v. infusion of 1-2 mg/minute for up to 24 hours. It is possible that in these concentrations frusemide is acting on the renal vasculature and increasing cortical blood flow. It should be stressed that the overall renal function is not improved by this technique as the urine passed still has low concentrations of urea and creatinine; but an increased excretion of water and potassium may be beneficial if cardiac failure and hyperkalaemia are life-threatening.

Conservative management

Once renal failure is established there is great danger in trying to force a diuresis by the continued intravenous administration of fluid. This only serves to produce dilutional hyponatraemia, fluid overload and cardiac failure. Instead, fluid intake should be carefully restricted to 500 ml plus the previous day's output.

A rising serum potassium level may produce fatal cardiac arrhythmias. If the level is above 6 mmol/litre it can be lowered by driving potassium into the cells using dextrose and insulin. The ratio of insulin to carbohydrate should be of the order of 3 g of carbohydrate to 1 unit of insulin, and a useful bolus injection would be 50 ml of 50% dextrose containing 8 units of soluble insulin.

The ECG changes of hyperkalaemia are of greater value than an absolute plasma concentration in assessing the potential danger due to a rising serum potassium. (Initially the T-wave becomes tented, but of greater significance is the widening of the QRS complex and the presence of ventricular ectopic beats.) An ion exchange resin (e.g. calcium resonium) can be given orally, but this regimen takes several hours before any noticeable effect is achieved.

Indications for dialysis

The main indication for dialysis, whether it be haemo- or peritoneal, is simply the presence of acute renal failure. Earlier texts advocated waiting until the patient was uraemic, acidotic and possibly overloaded with fluid before dialysis was suggested. Hyperkalaemia and fluid overload remain the indications for urgent dialysis, but it is now felt that there is little point in waiting until the patient is unwell before dialysis is commenced. The prognosis will be improved if the patient's clinical condition can be kept as stable as possible, and supportive dialysis should therefore be started as soon as a diuretic challenge has failed.

Wherever possible it is advisable for the patient to be transferred to a specialist renal unit. The technical procedure of dialysis and general clinical care, both need expertise and careful control if the patient is to be given the best chance of survival.

Supportive dialysis

The techniques of haemodialysis, haemofiltration and peritoneal dialysis are described in Chapter 5.

When fluid overload and pulmonary oedema are major problems, then haemofiltration can remove fluid quickly at a rate of 1-2 litres/hour. Then, if required, a short period of haemodialysis can be performed to reduce the levels of potassium, urea, etc. (The progress of a patient who was haemodialized is shown in Fig. 3.2 see p. 28.) Peritoneal dialysis is also excellent for removing fluid (Fig. 3.3 see p. 29) and correcting hyperkalacmia, but the poor clearances and risk of infection often limit its long-term value.

There is little doubt that daily haemodialysis for 4 hours to reduce the elevated potassium, urea and creatinine, combined with a period of haemofiltration to remove fluid in order to create a 'space' for nutrition, is the ideal form of treatment.

Early dialysis is essential to keep the patient as fit as possible but, despite early treatment, complications often occur.

Complications

Infection

The immune response is dampened in renal failure and patients are prone to infection. The normal signs of infection may be masked as the white cell count may remain normal and the patient apyrexial.

Anaemia

Owing to haemolysis and decreased red cell production, anaemia will develop within days from the onset of renal failure. Blood transfusion may be indicated if the haemoglobin drops to extremely low levels, but repeated transfusion has little value as the transfused cells will be rapidly broken down.

CNS disturbance

Electrolyte imbalance and the toxic metabolites that accumulate may produce a prolonged period of unconsciousness. Apart from frequent dialysis and supportive measures, there are no specific steps to be taken.

28 *Acute renal failure*

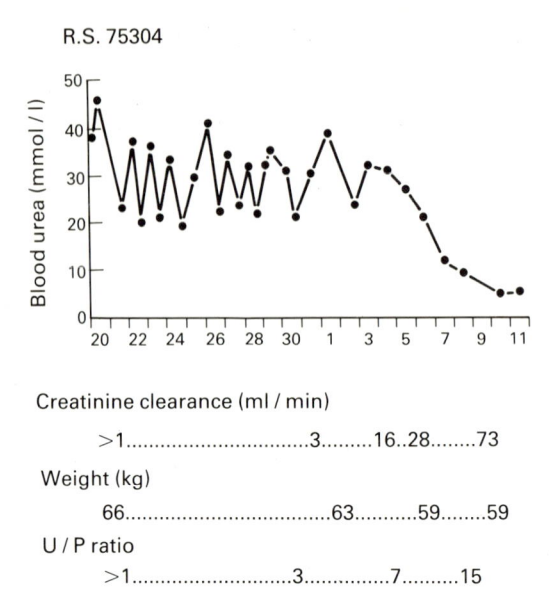

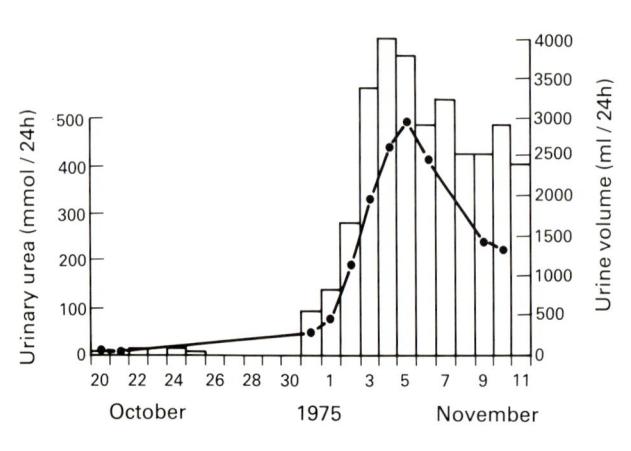

R.S. 75304

Creatinine clearance (ml / min)
>1..................................3.........16..28........73
Weight (kg)
66.................................63...........59........59
U / P ratio
>1..............................3...............7..........15

Fig. 3.2 Acute renal failure following open heart surgery. The sharp drops in blood urea represent periods of haemodialysis.

Hypertension

The patient with acute renal failure occasionally becomes hypertensive, a condition that can be sustained or may only occur during periods of haemodialysis. Routine treatment in the form of a beta-blocking drug plus a peripheral vasodilator is often extremely beneficial, and the combination of propranolol and hydralazine is often used. If the pressure rises abruptly to

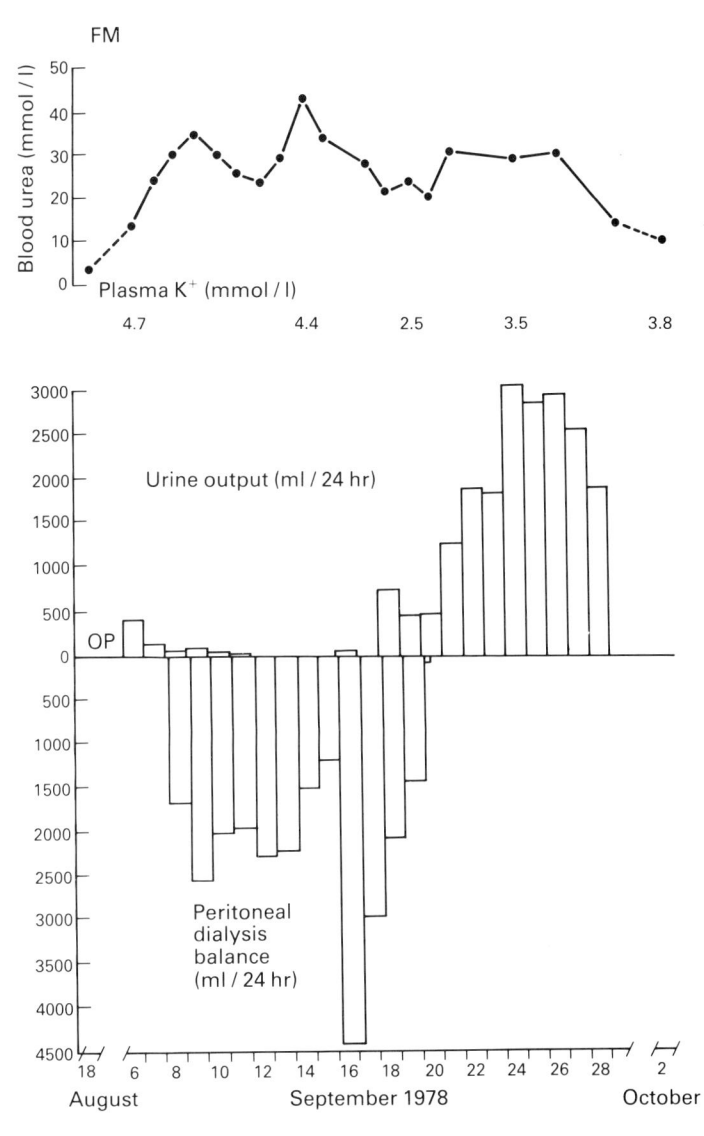

Fig. 3.3 Acute renal failure following cardiac surgery in a child, successfully managed with peritoneal dialysis.

dangerous levels during haemodialysis, then the combined alpha- and beta-adrenergic blocking drug labetalol can be given intravenously. Sodium and water retention may be a factor in producing hypertension, and in these cases the removal of fluid by ultrafiltration may be required (see Chapter 8).

General clinical management

Fluid and electrolyte balance

During the anuric period daily adjustments will have to be made to the fluid intake. Account should be taken of the fluid removed during dialysis, any urine produced, and insensible loss. In cases of polyuric renal failure the additional fluid will, of course, be given, and where necessary the urinary losses of electrolytes – mainly sodium and potassium – may need to be actively replaced. The patient's weight is an excellent guide to fluid balance; in the anuric catabolic phase a slight daily loss is to be expected, as account must be taken of the removal by dialysis of the water produced by metabolism.

Nutrition

Adequate calories must be given in the form of carbohydrates and lipids, which may be given intravenously in the early stages. If and when the patient's condition improves a 40–60 g protein diet is often well tolerated.

There is little point in administering large quantities of amino acids intravenously, since during the catabolic phase they will just serve to elevate the blood urea. There is little evidence that they can be actively incorporated into tissue and muscle until the anabolic phase is reached.

Drug administration

The pharmacokinetics of any drug administered must be clearly understood. In those cases in which the drug is solely eliminated by glomerular filtration (such as the aminoglycosides and digoxin) the dosage must be reduced. Wherever possible, drugs that are known to be nephrotoxic should be avoided.

The recovery phase

The period of anuria may last several days or may extend to 4–6 weeks. In the young patient with previously normal kidneys, the urine flow, once started, usually increases rapidly until 24-hour volumes of 2–3 litres are achieved. During this diuretic phase the tubules are unresponsive to antidiuretic hormone, and careful fluid and electrolyte control is still required. The urinary losses of sodium and potassium in particular may be considerable and will require accurate replacement.

Although in some cases the glomerular filtration rate may within weeks return to an almost normal level, the prognosis is not always good. When acute renal failure is associated with severe trauma (such as with major cardiac surgery or burns), the complications of the underlying condition are often fatal.

Acute tubular dysfunction is a potentially reversible situation. Supportive measures are justified as the fortunate patient may return to a normal life not requiring any specific therapy or dietary restriction.

4

Chronic renal failure

The clinical presentation and management of patients with severely reduced renal function can best be understood from a knowledge of the pathophysiology. In many instances careful, conservative treatment will maintain a reasonable standard of life until the glomerular filtration rate is approaching 15 ml/minute or less, at which point a decision has to be taken whether the patient is suitable for maintenance haemodialysis and/or transplantation.

Fortunately there is considerable reserve of renal function. About three-quarters has to be lost before significant nitrogen retention occurs and the patient develops symptoms. Patients may present complaining of general malaise, nausea and vomiting, and as part of the routine investigations the blood urea and creatinine are found to be raised. The appetite is often poor, there is a nasty taste in the mouth, and because of the accompanying anaemia the patients are often listless and complain of early fatigue on exercise. With further diminution in function normal sodium and water homeostasis deteriorates and an expansion of the circulating blood volume produces both peripheral and pulmonary oedema. The latter is, in some cases, the factor producing an acute illness. Systemic hypertension is often present and this will aggravate any cardiac failure associated with fluid overload.

One of the early changes associated with a reduction in renal function is loss of the ability to produce a concentrated or dilute urine, and polyuria and polydipsia result. The severe metabolic upset associated with uraemia may produce a peripheral neuropathy, and paraesthesiae are often present, especially in the lower limbs.

Aetiology

The renal tract can be involved in many disease processes, any of which may produce total renal failure. However, the common causes (with percentages) are:

Glomerulonephritis (40)
Pyelonephritis (20)
Cystic disease (10)
Hypertension (10)

Diabetes mellitus (5)
Drug nephropathy (3)
Remainder, including amyloid, oxalosis and unknown (12)

These figures only provide a general view of the problem, and patients may present in several categories. For example, diabetes is probably the commonest cause of chronic renal failure worldwide, for the patients are often recorded as having hypertension or infective problems. Some recorded statistics only relate to those patients taken on for maintenance dialysis, and since not all patients are suitable for dialysis some never appear in patient surveys.

Clinical assessment

History and examination
These should follow the scheme outlined in Chapter 1, with particular reference to the state of nutrition, hypertension and cardiac failure.

Routine ward testing of urine
This should include bacterial culture and examination of urine deposit.

Blood and urine biochemistry
It is necessary to measure the creatinine clearance, 24-hour protein excretion, pH and uric acid status. An accurate measure of the GFR, even when this is reduced, can be obtained by the isotopic method.

Imaging
A plain abdominal X-ray with tomography to assess renal size can be followed by ultrasound if needed. An IVU using isotonic contrast media with no previous dehydration will also provide measures of renal size and cortical width and will display any obstruction to the collecting system. Ultrasound, prograde (antegrade) and retrograde pyelograms may be required if obstruction is suspected (see Chapter 2). Renal scintigraphy will provide both anatomical information and a measure of function of each kidney separately (as well as of both overall) (see Chapter 1).

Plasma calcium, phosphate and alkaline phosphatase levels, along with hand, skull and spinal X-rays, are required to detect early forms of renal osteodystrophy (see Figs. 4.1 and 4.2).

Renal biopsy
This should be performed if the diagnosis is in doubt, especially when the kidneys are large and not obstructed. Amyloid and multiple myeloma may be present.

Clinical assessment 33

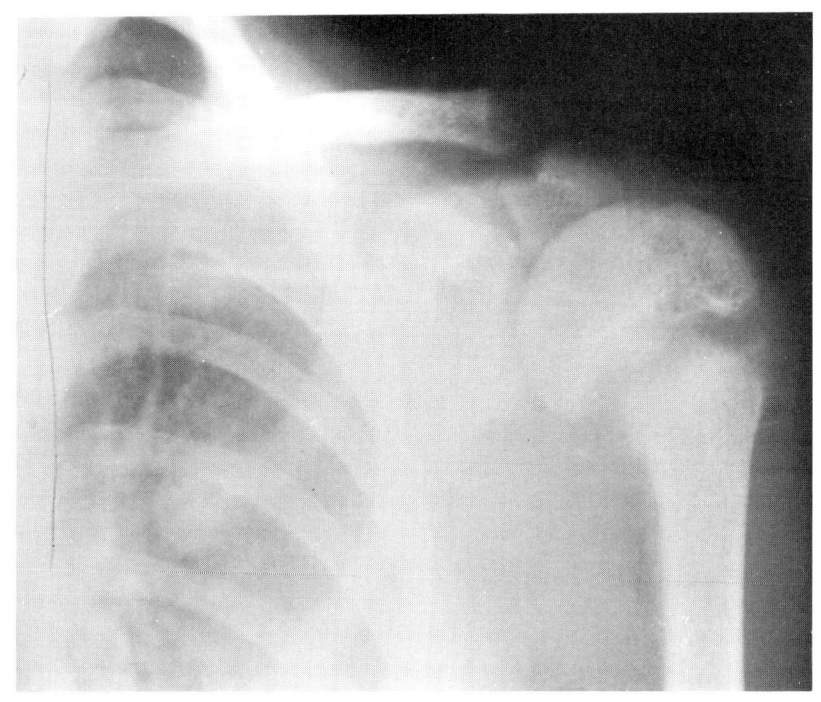

Fig. 4.1 Delayed fusion of the upper end of the humerus and clavicular erosion in a young adult with renal osteodystrophy.

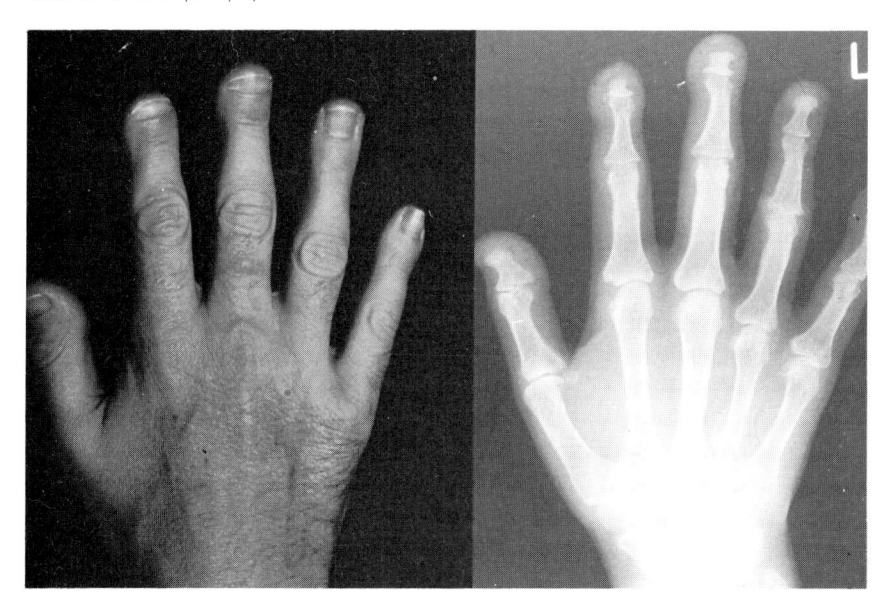

Fig. 4.2 Erosion of the terminal phalanges producing pseudo-clubbing in a patient with severe long-standing renal osteodystrophy.

Chest X-ray and ECG

Heart size, pleural effusion and the state of the left ventricle can be assessed from the X-ray and ECG. A more accurate cardiac assessment would involve isotopic scintigraphy and echo cardiography.

Management

Treatment of any underlying cause is important, but so often when renal function is severely reduced treatment is ineffective or even inappropriate. If obstruction has been excluded as a cause, specific areas of management will be related to the underlying pathophysiology. These will now be discussed in some detail.

Nitrogen retention

The three main nitrogenous compounds excreted by the kidney are urea, creatinine and uric acid (Hladky and Rink, Chapter 11).

Urea

This is the end result of protein catabolism taking place in the liver, so that production with a normal liver function will depend on the catabolic rate and the dietary intake of protein. Urea is removed by the kidney primarily by filtration, with little evidence of tubular secretion (Hladky and Rink, pp. 99–101).

The relationship of the plasma level to the GFR is described in Chapter 1. From Fig. 1.1 it may be seen that a low protein intake will lower the blood urea. This drop in plasma concentration may reduce nausea and vomiting – a gain in patient comfort that is valuable but which should not be at the cost of poor nutrition. Even at low levels of function the patient remains in nitrogen balance, and it is essential that adequate protein – along with sufficient calories, often in the form of fat and carbohydrates – should be given to prevent malnutrition.

In the 1950s diets were carefully constructed to contain the essential amino acids (the so-called Giovanetti diet); but with dialysis facilities becoming more readily available, strict protein restriction has largely been discontinued. More recent evidence suggests that early protein restriction may indeed slow down the rate of functional deterioration, the rationale being that the high osmotic load presented to the remaining nephrons as a result of a normal diet accentuates glomerular damage – hyperfiltration nephropathy. Even if this is true, it will be difficult to persuade the asymptomatic patient with a GFR of 50–60 ml/minute to adhere to a strict dietary regime.

The essential amino acids have a carbon chain that cannot be synthesized, but attempts have been made to provide their keto-analogues, thus reducing the nitrogen intake. This idea, although attractive, has not gained general acceptance. Patients are therefore given a 40–60 g protein diet when symptomatic, and their future replacement policy is discussed. If, for any reason, dialysis or transplantation is not appropriate, then to limit first-class protein to one main meal in the day is a humane compromise.

Uraemic symptoms are not produced solely by an elevated urea or creatinine, as many other metabolic end-products such as phenols and acid radicals accumulate in renal failure. These as yet unidentified compounds are given the general term of 'middle molecules' – their molecular weights, 500–5000 daltons, fall between those of the small molecules such as urea, which are easily removed by dialysis, and those of the large proteinaceous molecules which are not cleared by this technique. The search continues to define these possible toxic substances.

Creatinine

This is the end-product of muscle metabolism. Owing to this solely endogenous source the plasma level is not influenced by diet or liver function, but it is dependent on the glomerular filtration rate and the muscle mass.

Creatinine clearance approximates closely to the glomerular filtration rate, and again, as with urea, the plasma concentration does not have a linear relationship with the glomerular filtration rate. Carefully measured plasma levels are, however, a useful guide for following changes in renal function; some clinicians prefer to plot the reciprocal value against time and use this plot to predict future levels of function.

Uric acid

Derived mainly from nuclear protein, this acid accumulates rapidly in the plasma when the glomerular filtration rate falls below 30 ml/minute. Synthesis can be reduced by a xanthine oxidase inhibitor such as allopurinol, but generally when high plasma levels are achieved dialysis will be indicated.

Sodium and water balance

Hladky and Rink (Chapter 14) describe the central role of renal sodium and water homeostasis in the maintenance of an adequate circulation. As the GFR falls the amount of filtered sodium falls, but the glomerular–tubular balance is maintained since the urinary loss of sodium is increased to keep the patient in sodium balance. The tubular compensating mechanisms are poorly understood, but they clearly involve reduced reabsorption of sodium by the proximal tubule. When single-figure clearances are reached, sodium retention may require dietary restriction to control hypertension and fluid overload. These often develop simultaneously.

Not all patients retain sodium. In some, excessive urinary losses may accompany the high urine flow rate that results from the obligatory solute load delivered to the tubules of the remaining nephrons. It is thought that the high tubular osmotic concentration coupled with the rapid transit time through the tubule limits sodium reabsorption. This explanation assumes that the reduced numbers of nephrons are physiologically normal and behave in a predictable fashion when faced with an increased amount of filtered solute – the 'intact nephron' hypothesis. It is clear that this is not the sole explanation since some tubules are damaged and the increased natriuresis represents tubular damage.

If excessive sodium loss is not replaced the circulating volume will fall, followed by hypotension and reduced renal perfusion, which will reduce the glomerular filtration rate even further. This downward spiral must be prevented by adequate sodium replacement. Salt added to food may suffice, but added supplements in the form of sodium bicarbonate may be required. The bicarbonate radical will help to correct the metabolic acidosis usually present at this level of function. However, reduction in ionized calcium with alkali therapy may precipitate muscle spasm and tetany.

As the GFR falls the ability to concentrate and dilute urine is lost, and its osmolality becomes fixed close to that of plasma at around 300 mosmol/kg. The inability to concentrate means that during periods when excess fluid is lost – for example, with vomiting and diarrhoea – the kidney cannot conserve fluid and inappropriately high volumes of urine are passed. Again, hypotension and poor renal perfusion may develop, thus aggravating an already impaired function. If the reduction is severe then acute upon chronic renal failure is the result. If the patient presents in time, fluid losses should be replaced, intravenously if necessary; and body weight, blood pressure, central venous pressure and tissue turgor are all guides to fluid replacement.

Diuretics such as frusemide and the thiazides will promote sodium and water loss even when renal function is reduced. Higher doses may be required to achieve an increased urine volume, which may be beneficial in some patients who have become oliguric. There is no improvement in function but the increased urine output does allow patients to drink more. However, diuretics must be used with care as excessive iatrogenic sodium and water losses may produce the previously described deterioration in function. They are useful to promote potassium loss when hyperkalaemia is a problem.

Potassium

This is predominantly an intracellular ion and the plasma level represents a small fraction of the total body content. The plasma level will rise in renal failure as urinary losses diminish and the acidosis associated with renal impairment forces potassium to leave the cell as hydrogen enters (Hladky and Rink, pp. 133–8). The slow elevation that occurs in chronic renal failure seems to provide some adaptation, since cardiac arrythmias are not as marked in these patients as they are in those who develop acute renal failure.

Avoidance of foods rich in potassium – such as fruit, chocolate, etc. – is the first stage in managing hyperkalaemia; this is followed by the use of diuretics. Ion-exchange resins and intravenous dextrose and insulin may be used as a holding procedure while dialysis is being instigated.

Metabolic acidosis

Renal acidification (Hladky and Rink, pp. 65–8, 85–91, Chapter 17) is reduced, so that the 100 mmol of hydrogen ion produced by a normal diet cannot be eliminated and systemic acidosis results. Either ammonia production is reduced or the proximal tubule cannot reabsorb the bulk of the filtered bicarbonate, and the inappropriate loss produces a constantly alkaline urine.

Long-term administration of oral sodium bicarbonate has only a minimal effect on the plasma pH. In any case, this treatment should be carried out with care as the additional sodium may precipitate cardiac failure and aggravate hypertension, and it may depress the ionized calcium fraction, producing muscle cramp and tetany.

Hypertension

Hypertension may develop, or its control become more difficult, when sodium and water retention occur (Hladky and Rink, Chapter 15). Dietary sodium restriction coupled with diuretic therapy may be adequate, but often it is not until the patient is dialysed or receives a functioning transplant that the hypertension is corrected. In some patients it is a loss of renal vasodilating substances such as prostaglandin that appears to be important, while in others the elevated pressure may be sustained by renal ischaemia, due either to a major vessel occlusion or to generalized parenchymal damage. If a major vessel stenosis is confirmed by angiography then it may be possible, using a balloon catheter, to dilate the vessel, improving blood flow and thereby abolishing the hypertension as well as possibly improving function. This procedure, known as percutaneous transluminal dilatation, has been used successfully in coronary vessels. (In addition, just as cardiologists are using argon lasers to correct coronary stenosis, it is possible that laser therapy will be used in other parts of the vascular tree with benefit.)

When generalized ischaemia is due to small vessel damage, mechanical intervention has no place. If the hypertension is difficult to control despite adequate dialysis, then a bilateral nephrectomy is indicated.

Calcium and phosphate

Disordered calcium and phosphate homeostasis is associated with bone disease. This occurs as renal function diminishes and, now that patients are kept alive by maintenance dialysis, more florid forms of bone pathology are being recognized. Several factors appear to be operating and the mechanisms are still the subject of research (Hladky and Rink, pp. 138–41). The following outline provides an understanding of therapy.

With a reduced glomerular filtration rate, phosphate excretion is diminished and the plasma level rises. Since the product of calcium and phosphate ion concentrations is fixed, calcium ion concentration in the plasma falls. Disordered vitamin D metabolism may also produce a lowered serum calcium since the kidney is the site for activation of this vitamin, producing its final active form, ^{1,25}dihydrocholicalciferol (DHCC). Vitamin D promotes calcium absorption from the gut, so that with a lack of the active compound the plasma levels fall owing to diminished gut absorption. The lowered serum calcium stimulates parathyroid hormone (PTH) production, which can be measured in the blood. However, with current techniques it is not certain whether the active, complete molecule, or only certain fragments of the amino-acid chain, is being measured.

The elevated PTH level will promote bone reabsorption by increased osteoblastic activity, and this can be demonstrated radiologically by the presence of periosteal erosions seen in the phalanges. The reabsorption may be so severe as to erode the terminal phalanges (Fig. 4.2 see p. 33). In some areas increased PTH activity is associated with osteosclerosis which appears radiologically as an increased bone density. It is almost certainly a lack of active vitamin D that produces osteomalacia, which appears as areas of decalcified bone. These may present on X-rays as discrete bands across the neck of a long bone (Looser's zones), or may appear as pseudofractures in long-standing cases. The presence of osteosclerosis and osteomalacia in the spine gives the characteristic banded appearance which has been graphically described as the 'rugger jersey spine'. It should be noted that osteomalacia is an extreme condition associated with long-standing disease, as well over 50 per cent of skeletal calcium has to be lost before it can be detected radiologically. Associated with osteomalacia is a myopathy that presents as painful muscles, a symptom that fortunately responds rapidly to vitamin D therapy.

This combined assault on the skeleton leads to deformity and pain and so should be prevented if at all possible. Plasma phosphate levels may be lowered by binding the dietary phosphate in the gut using aluminium hydroxide. An active form of vitamin D, 1-α-dihydroxy-cholicalciferol, can be given, often with calcium supplements, to maintain calcium levels within the normal range. Guides to the success of treatment would be radiological improvement and a reduction in the plasma concentration of alkaline phosphatase, an enzyme present in bone which is increased during osteoblastic activity. The value of early and even prophylactic treatment is not certain; but it is clear that prolonged parathyroid stimulation produces *secondary* hyperparathyroidism, which may cause the gland to maintain increased levels of parathyroid hormone production even when the stimuli have been removed by therapy (*tertiary* hyperparathyroidism). In such cases the autonomous glands may have to be removed surgically. Normally only one-eighth of one gland is left, but this is usually adequate to maintain the plasma calcium within the normal range. If hypocalcaemia develops, however, vitamin D and oral calcium supplementation may be required. There is a risk that renal function will deteriorate during this procedure, but it is a risk that has to be taken.

Osteoporosis may also occur in renal failure, but the aetiology of this reduction of bone mass which histologically appears normal is uncertain.

Anaemia

Severe anaemia is a late complication of renal failure and unfortunately there is no effective treatment. Diminished erythropoietin production by the kidney limits the maturation of red cells from bone marrow precursors. Elevated urea and other toxins that accumulate in the blood are a poor environment for the red cell and the lifespan is greatly reduced from the normal 120 days. Dietary deficiency of haematinics, and gastrointestinal blood loss which is secondary to uraemic gastritis and enterocolitis, are contributory factors.

The presence of severe anaemia clearly aggravates cardiac failure and angina and slows postoperative wound healing; it is therefore disappointing that no satisfactory treatment is available. A course of oral iron and folic acid may help some patients, but it is only after successful transplantation that the anaemia is corrected.

Glucose metabolism

Glucose metabolism is not markedly altered. In uraemia insulin is less effective, but the breakdown of insulin by the kidney is reduced. These factors tend to cancel out, but some diabetics find that as renal failure progresses, insulin requirements fall.

Infection

Severe infection is common in advanced failure owing to dampening down of the immune system.

Substitution therapy

Once chronic renal failure has been confirmed the foregoing conservative measures can be employed with benefit to forestall the time of substitution therapy. Once the creatinine clearance falls to below 30 ml/minute then a decision should be taken as to the appropriate form of long-term substitution therapy.

5
Dialysis

The principles of dialysis are applied from the field of chemical engineering as well as from clinical nephrology. When two solutions are separated by a semi-permeable membrane, permeant particles will move across the membrane from a higher to a lower concentration. Since membranes have various pore sizes, some will allow only small molecules to pass while others with a larger pore size will be more permeable. This selective passive diffusion across a semi-permeable membrane is known as dialysis.

In the support of patients with acute or chronic renal failure, blood must pass on one side of a semi-permeable membrane while a dialysate solution passes on the other side In *peritoneal dialysis* the patient's own peritoneum is regarded as the semi-permeable membrane and the dialysate is run in and out of the peritoneal cavity. This procedure can be used for acute renal failure, and it has recently been used for the long-term management of chronic renal failure and referred to as chronic ambulatory peritoneal dialysis (CAPD). For *haemodialysis*, however, an extracorporeal blood circuit is required to pass the patient's blood in contact with an artificial semi-permeable membrane, with the dialysate passing on the opposite side in a contraflow fashion. Once again this technique can be used for both acute and chronic renal failure, and an outline of the procedures involved with the relative advantages and disadvantages will be of value to the student. At this stage a detailed technical account is unnecessary.

Haemodialysis

Arterial blood has to pass across a semi-permeable membrane of suitable area and composition to achieve adequate dialysis. The increased area required to allow suitable diffusion is currently achieved either by arranging the membrane in a series of flat plates between which the dialysate can flow, or by producing the membrane in the form of hollow fibres (Fig. 5.1). With this configuration areas of between 0.5 and 2.00 m^2 can be achieved, with the standard size for most adults being 1.5 m^2. Dialysate of suitable chemical composition is pumped in the direction opposite to the blood flow. The chemical composition of the dialysate can vary, but a typical composition expressed in mmol/litre is: Na 130-135, K 0-3.5, Ca 1.4-1.8, Mg 0.25, Cl 95-100, lactate or bicarbonate 40, glucose 0-10. The osmolality is not fixed and can be varied

Haemodialysis 41

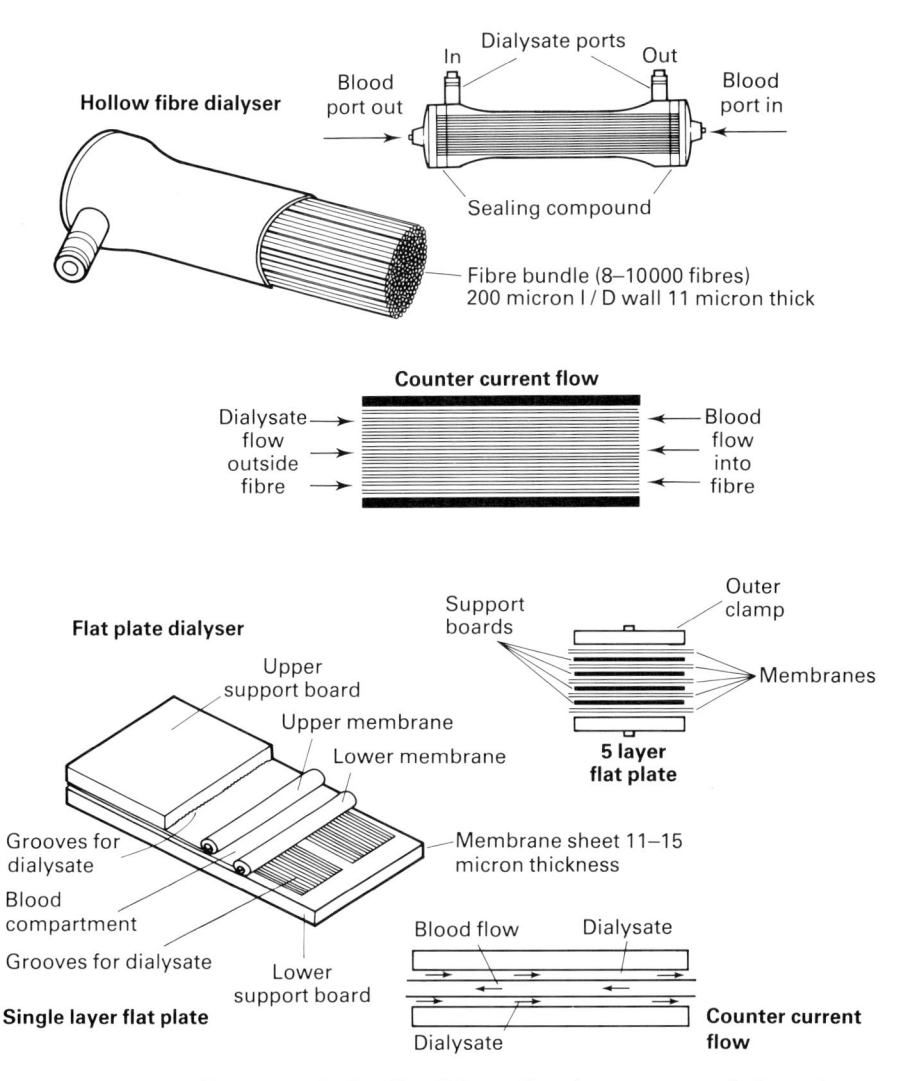

Fig. 5.1 Diagrams of flat plate and hollow fibre dialysers. Note the arrangements for increasing the surface area of the dialyser membrane.

according to the patient's needs. A high osmolality may be required in order to remove water by osmosis and is often achieved by raising the glucose concentration.

The elevated plasma urea, creatinine, phosphate and uric acid diffuse into the dialysate and are removed, while bicarbonate or lactate diffuse in the opposite direction into the patient's circulation, achieving temporary correction of his or her acidosis.

Early membranes were made of Cellophane, but most modern dialysers

42 Dialysis

incorporate the cellulose derivative cuprophane. It will be seen later that more highly permeable membranes have been developed, allowing large volumes of fluid to be removed quickly in a process known as haemofiltration.

To achieve satisfactory exchange the pressure and flow of blood and dialysate are critical. The rate of pure water removal across the membrane can be increased either by increasing the osmotic pressure of the dialysate, by employing the principle of osmosis, or by altering the pressure gradient across the membrane. The latter can be achieved by increasing the pressure in the blood compartment or by producing a negative pressure on the dialysate side. Whichever of these techniques is employed, the removal of the excess fluid is called *ultrafiltration*.

It is not surprising that during dialysis, with its major shifts of fluid and electrolytes (particularly potassium), circulatory changes occur. Cardiac arrhythmias (commonly ventricular ectopic beats), are associated with shifts of potassium, while volume changes may be associated with profound hypotension. This may require reinfusion of saline and plasma into the patient's circulation. Muscle cramps are a disturbing complaint, especially in those patients with chronic renal failure requiring supportive dialysis two to three times a week for periods of 4–6 hours at a time. Owing to the high metabolic rate in acute renal failure, daily periods of dialysis of up to 3–4 hours are required. The complications of dialysis may be prevented or significantly reduced if the ultrafiltration is separated from the period of chemical dialysis.

Access to the circulation in patients with acute renal failure is either by the insertion of Teflon cannulae into a peripheral artery and vein (Fig. 5.2), with the two cannulae being bridged with a silastic tube to maintain the circulation when not in use, or by cannulation of a central vein with a double lumen cannula. Infection, thrombosis and haemorrhage are obvious complications of both techniques. For long-term access an arteriovenous fistula is created, often at the wrist, by side-to-side anastomosis of the radial artery to the cephalic vein. When the veins are subject to arterial pressure and flow they dilate and the walls become thickened (Fig. 5.3), allowing the easy introduction of cannulae to remove and return blood to the circulation. Once established, an a–v fistula can be used for many years, but occasionally aneurysm formation or gradual stenosis limits its use. If the orifice between artery and vein is too large then

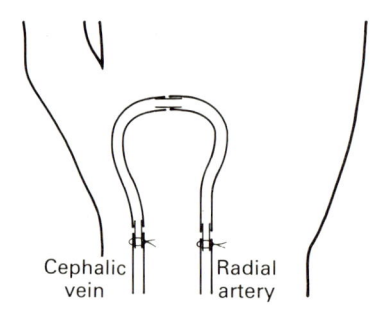

Fig. 5.2 Diagram of arteriovenous shunt at the wrist, used for acute renal failure. Teflon tips are sutured into the radial artery and cephalic vein.

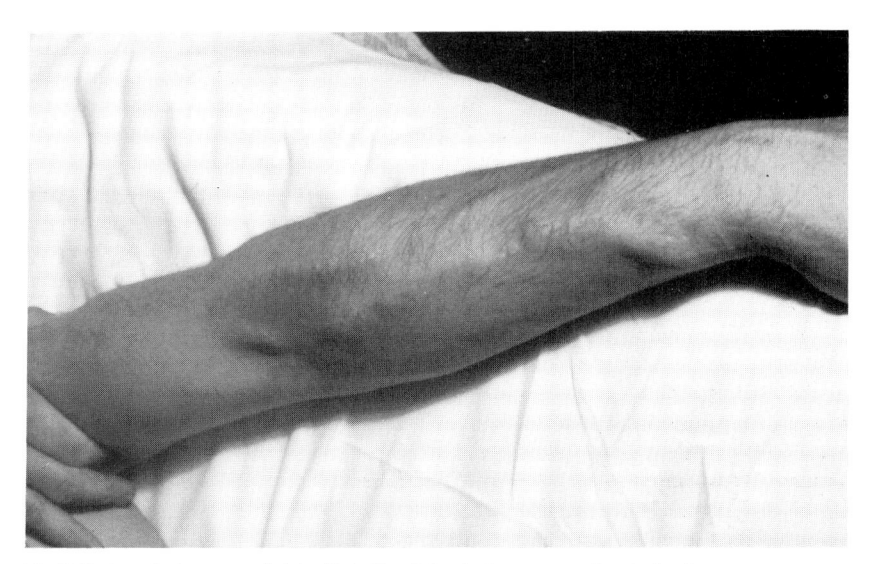

Fig. 5.3 An arteriovenous fistula. Note the distended venous system in the forearm.

considerable flows develop, and this may lead to high-output cardiac failure, a condition obviously made worse by the pre-existing anaemia. When a–v fistulae fail and no vessels for anastomosis are available, then an artificial material such as Dacron or processed animal veins may be used to join the artery and vein, with direct cannulation of the artificial material. These are prone to infection and often have a short life.

Haemofiltration

A recent development using a highly permeable membrane made of polyacronlile nitrite is proving useful in the management of acute renal failure. The membrane is made in the form of hollow fibres.

Often the patient's own blood pressure is adequate to perfuse the fibres and produce a filtrate of up to 1–2 litres/hour. If the patient's pressure is not sufficient then an occlusive roller pump may be placed in the circuit.

Vascular access can be via an a–v shunt or by central venous cannulation. The blood is heparinized before it is passed through the membrane, and the fluid that is removed has the same constituents as blood except for protein and cells. Large volumes of filtrate are removed containing the high plasma concentrations of potassium, urea, creatinine, etc., and a replacement fluid containing the electrolytes in normal concentrations with no potassium is used.

If, say, 1 litre of filtrate is removed from the patient per hour, then this allows 900 ml of fluid to be replaced. The bulk of the replacement fluid has the constitution mentioned, but the remainder can allow adequate parenteral nutrition in the form of glucose, amino acids and lipid. If the patient is in cardiac failure or severe circulatory overload, then much less fluid can be replaced, allowing a negative balance to develop. As large volumes per hour are

44 *Dialysis*

lost, careful management of the replacement fluid is essential if hyper- or hypovolaemia are to be prevented. Instead of haemofiltration being limited to 3–4 hours per day, it can be a continuous process and adequate clearances can be achieved, allowing the technique to be used for several days (if not weeks) with the critically ill patient. With this more gentle, continuous process the circulation remains more stable and hypotension and arrhythmias are usually avoided.

At present in specialist renal units a mixture of haemofiltration and conventional dialysis is often used.

Peritoneal dialysis

Although this procedure does not require expensive and complicated equipment and can therefore be used in a general hospital ward, it can, in inexperienced hands, produce serious clinical complications.

The patient's peritoneum acts as the semi-permeable membrane. Dialysate at body temperature is introduced into the abdominal cavity in order that exchange may take place between the blood in the mesenteric vessels of the peritoneum and the dialysate fluid (Fig. 5.4). Obviously the area of exchange is fixed, but where the metabolic rate is not high the clearance of creatinine and urea are usually adequate. This is especially true in children, for whom the ratio of the peritoneal area to body mass is high.

The clearance of urea and creatinine may not be adequate for prolonged treatment; but potassium and fluid removal are often very easily achieved, and so this technique may be used to correct dangerous hyperkalaemia and fluid

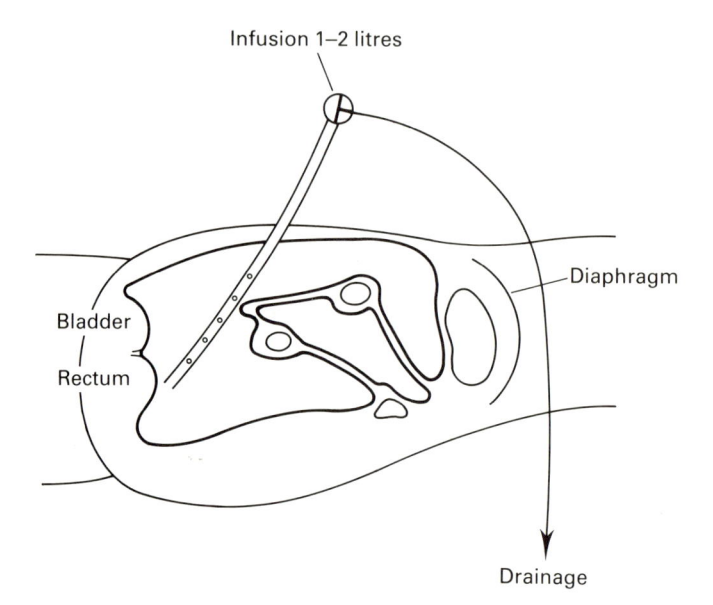

Fig. 5.4 Diagram of peritoneal dialysis showing the cannula in position and the large area of peritoneum available for exchange.

Table 5.1 Composition of peritoneal dialysis solutions expressed in mmol/litre

Na	Cl	Lactate	Ca	Mg	Glucose (%)
130	90	45	1.8	0.7	1.36
140	101	45	1.8	0.7	1.36
140	101	45	1.8	0.7	3.86

K^+ can be added as required.

overload and, as a holding measure, is perfectly adequate while awaiting specialist help.

The composition of the peritoneal fluid can vary, and Table 5.1 provides the composition of the three commonly used solutions. Additional potassium may be added to prevent hypokalaemia, and if hyperglycaemia is a problem insulin can be added to the solution – an excellent mode of administration since it passes directly into the portal circulation.

Membrane transport may diminish with time because of the onset of peritonitis, due either to bacterial infection of yeasts, or secondary to chemical damage – a condition known as chemical peritonitis. Protein may leak from the blood into the dialysate; if this leakage is excessive, protein replacement into the patient's circulation will have to be commenced. Similarly, large volumes of fluid may be removed and the two factors taken together may produce profound hypovolaemia and hypotension.

This approach has been used for both acute and chronic renal failure, and a brief outline of the two techniques will now be given.

Acute peritoneal dialysis

In patients with acute renal failure a temporary, rigid catheter is inserted just below the umbilicus in the mid-line and directed down towards the pelvis. Strict asepsis is required. After local anaesthesia, a small incision is made to facilitate catheter insertion, which is also made easier if the patient is able consciously to contract the recti. If the patient is unconscious or paralysed the use of a fine needle to fill the peritoneal cavity with 2 litres of dialysate will make insertion of the large catheter safer, as bowel perforation is a possible complication of insertion. A deep purse-string suture stabilizes the catheter and prevents leakage.

Warmed dialysate with 500 units of heparin per litre should be run into the peritoneal cavity and then rapidly drained. Once dialysis is established then the heparin can be discontinued. Depending on the size of the patient, 1- or 2-litre cycles can be employed, but a larger volume may elevate the diaphragm, embarrass respiration and cause respiratory distress. As a general principle rapid exchanges are employed, with the fluid being run in as quickly as possible, left to dwell for 20 or 30 minutes and then drained, the whole cycle taking about 1 hour. Experience with individual patients may show that a longer dwell time of up to 1-2 hours may be beneficial; but if fluid removal and the lowering of an elevated serum potassium are the major considerations, then initially rapid exchanges should be used.

At the onset of dialysis the drainage may be bloodstained, but usually with time this will clear. Bacterial and fungal infections remain a problem, and both intraperitoneal and systemic antibiotics may be needed. Care should be taken if the aminoglycosides are used as, from an inflamed peritoneum, the absorption is considerable and toxic plasma levels may be attained.

The peritoneum is sensitive to stretch, and rapid infusion may produce pain; the addition of local anaesthetic is usually unrewarding, but slower infusion of dialysate, carefully adjusted to body temperature, usually helps.

Recent abdominal surgery is not an absolute contraindication, but dialysate may leak through the recent incision. If the diaphragm has been opened during thoracic surgery, the passage of dialysate through the diaphragm into the chest can present a serious infective risk. The presence of infection is not a reason for stopping as peritoneal lavage is an accepted form of treatment for peritonitis.

This form of dialysis can be continued for many weeks if adequate clearances are obtained, or used initially as a holding operation before haemodialysis can be performed.

Chronic ambulatory peritoneal dialysis (CAPD)

Peritoneal dialysis has been used intermittently since the 1960s as supportive treatment for patients with end-stage renal failure. Rigid catheters were used, patients were often confined to hospital for long periods, and inevitably sepsis occurred.

When soft, pliable catheters were used and inserted under direct vision through a small laparotomy, with the catheter tubing tunnelled through the skin, chronic ambulatory peritoneal dialysis as a technique was born. Since then greater numbers of patients have benefited from this technique, and no longer is it the case that it is acceptable only for those who are unsuitable for haemodialysis.

Two litres of dialysate are used and four exchanges are made in a 24-hour period. After the dialysate has been run in, the empty plastic bag is rolled and remains attached to the cannula until the abdomen is drained into the same container; then the bag is removed and discarded. Strict aseptic techniques are used and, of the four exchanges, often one or two employ hypertonic solutions to achieve satisfactory fluid removal.

Infection remains the major problem. Careful patient training and dedicated microbiology are essential. There is little if any place for prophylactic antibiotics, but intraperitoneal regimens using gentamicin, metronidazole and the cephalosporins are often effective. If infection persists then the catheter must be removed, and the abdomen rested while the patient is haemodialysed for a period of 4-6 weeks.

With time, in a few patients the peritoneum becomes sclerosed and clearances are inadequate. Other complications – such as scrotal oedema, poor drainage, and fluid finding its way through the diaphragm into the pleural cavity – pose occasional problems.

There are, however, definite advantages. The continuous process means that there are no major changes in the plasma biochemistry which are associated with short periods of haemodialysis. These acute changes in weight, blood pressure and biochemistry often make the patient unwell for several hours, but with the steady state produced by CAPD the procedure is far better tolerated by the patient. The clearances achieved, along with adequate fluid removal, mean that the patient can have greater dietary freedom and often a free fluid intake; and, because the procedure is carried out in the home or place of work, there is also freedom of travel and mobility. There is some evidence, too, that patients undergoing CAPD have a higher haemoglobin and there is special benefit to the diabetic patient in whom vascular access is a major problem. Insulin can be given intraperitoneally, giving a smoother level of blood sugar.

All dialysis techniques for chronic renal failure are expensive and demand a high degree of patient compliance. It is hoped that the patient will be suitable for transplantation, as this means the patient has a chance of achieving a far superior quality of life.

6

Transplantation

All organ transplantations require suppression of the recipient's response to the introduction of foreign antigenic material that is mainly protein in nature. Without treatment the body will reject the organ by a combination of cellular invasion and circulating antibody. Blood vessels are damaged and the resultant ischaemia adds to the tissue damage produced by a cellular infiltration of immune competent lymphocytes.

With the development of the 6-Mercaptopurine (6-MP) derivatives in the 1960s the first real chance of successful immunosuppression was taken and renal transplantation began in earnest, using azathioprine (a safer derivative of 6-MP) and steroid as the standard form of treatment. Lymph duct cannulation, radiotherapy to the graft and host were tried, and much later plasma exchange was performed in an attempt to remove circulating immune complexes. This technique has not gained wide acceptance but, with the introduction of cyclosporin A and the use of antilymphocytic globulin, the chance of graft survival has increased.

The aim is to transplant kidneys into patients with chronic renal failure, as the quality of life is then vastly superior to that possible with any form of maintenance dialysis.

Here, details of surgery and postoperative management will follow an outline of the appropriate immunology.

Immunology

Although an understanding of the immunological principles of transplantation is vital to successful clinical management, there is not the space here to cover this important subject in great detail. The reading list will allow the student to cover the subject in greater depth.

The foreign antigens that provide tissue identity are glycoproteins fixed in the cell surface, and when a kidney is transplanted these glycoproteins are taken up on the surface of circulating dendritic cells and macrophages. These are regarded as messenger cells, as they present the antigen to the helper T-lymphocytes found in lymph nodes and bone marrow. Once stimulated these cells, via the production of chemical messengers called lymphokines, activate the B-lymphocytes to produce antibody and the circulating T-lymphocytes

Clinical signs of rejection damage

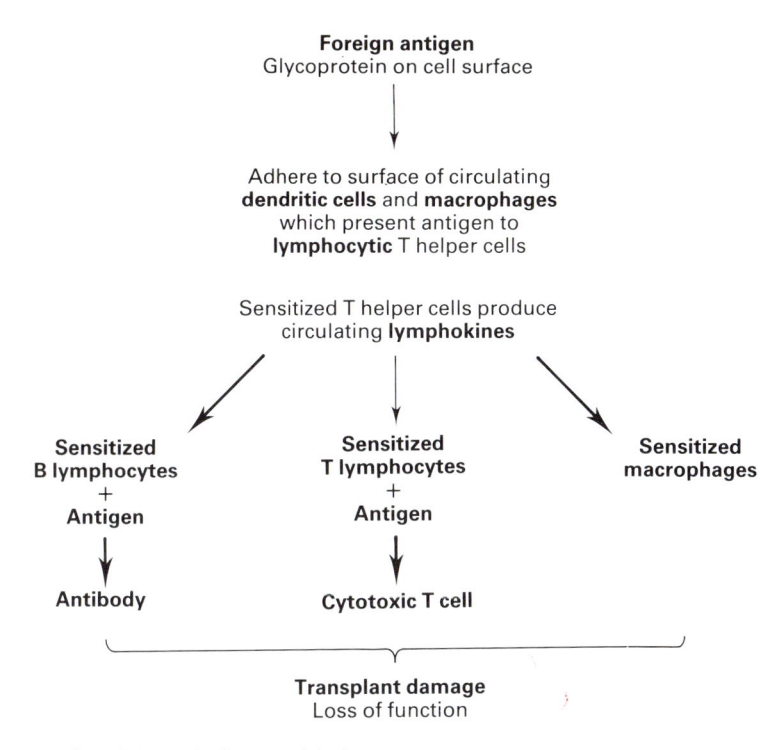

Fig. 6.1 Schematic diagram of the immune response.

assume cytotoxic potential, i.e. they are transformed into 'killer cells'. Circulating macrophages are stimulated and these may be responsible for tissue damage within the graft. These events are outlined in Fig. 6.1.

Clinical signs of rejection damage

Rejection damage can occur as soon as the vascular anastomoses are complete (*hyperacute rejection*), or during the first three months (*acute rejection*), or beyond three months (*chronic rejection*). The pathology of the three groups is as follows.

Hyperacute rejection

Instead of the kidney becoming pink and firm when blood flow is returned, the transplant becomes blue and flaccid within minutes. With light microscopy it is seen that the small capillaries within the glomeruli and around the tubules are swollen with clumps of red cells. Haemorrhage is seen in the interstitial areas, and later the vessels demonstrate fibrinoid damage within the walls. The lumina are then occluded by thrombi. This situation is produced by the presence in the patient's circulation of preformed antibodies, possibly as the result of pregnancy, previous blood transfusions or an earlier failed transplant. There is no successful treatment and it is for this reason that, as will be seen later, screening is undertaken to ensure as far as possible that there are no harmful circulating antibodies.

Acute rejection

This occurs commonly in the first two months and often the first episode occurs within 14 days. The kidney appears swollen and plum-coloured owing to venous congestion and oedema. When antibody-initiated damage predominates, vascular changes are seen as the capillaries are occluded by platelet aggregates and fibrin thrombi. The damage produced by killer T-cells leads to separation of the tubules by oedema and a parenchymal infiltrate of cells. If haemorrhage is present then the prognosis is poor. Often a mixed picture is seen. Biopsy assessment is essential because, as will be seen later, a distinction between rejection, acute tubular necrosis and drug toxicity – in particular due to cyclosporin – is required.

Chronic rejection

The kidney is once more large and the damage is mainly mediated by circulating antibodies: the glomeruli are smaller and the basement membrane may be thickened and appear wrinkled with, on occasions, complete hyalinization and total glomerular destruction. The lumina of interlobular and arcuate vessels along with the glomerular arterioles are narrowed by thickening of the wall owing to cell proliferation, swelling and disintegration which produce distal ischaemia and reduction in renal function.

Measures to prevent rejection damage

Two main approaches are employed: transplantation of kidneys that are antigenically as similar to the recipient as possible; and the use of immunosuppressive drugs.

Tissue matching

The antigens on the surface of all cells are also found on the surface of circulating lymphocytes and, with the use of specific antisera, it is possible in the laboratory to identify most of the antigens. As it is convenient to use circulating lymphocytes the system is known as the HLA (human lymphocyte antigens) system.

It is known that the genes responsible for reproduction of the HLA antigens are to be found on the 6th chromosome. Various areas or loci on the chromosome are responsible for the transmission of various sets of antigens. It is possible to isolate in some patients very clearly what types of antigen are associated with three main loci (A, B and D), and with knowledge of both donor and recipient careful matching can be achieved. With close matching the results of the graft and patient survival are improved, although with the use of cyclosporin it appears that accurate matching is no longer quite so important.

The problem of hyperacute rejection has been mentioned, and it is important to ensure that there are no circulating, preformed antibodies in the recipient that could react with the transplant antigens. A laboratory-based test can be employed for this purpose using the white cells from the donor and serum from the recipient. The donor leucocytes must remain viable in the presence of the recipient's serum. If this direct cross-match test is negative, and there is a successful degree of tissue matching, then the transplant can proceed. Clearly at the outset blood group compatibility will have been secured.

Immunosuppression

Azathioprine

This is a safer derivative of 6-MP. It is now widely used and for several years it was the standard immunosuppressor along with steroid. Apart from its general anti-inflammatory properties it also prevents lymphocytic proliferation. It can cause bone marrow depression and rarely anaemia and liver damage.

Steroids

Steroids are used mainly for their general anti-inflammatory properties, but they also reduce the synthesis of antibody. Maintenance therapy is with oral prednisolone, with intravenous methylprednisolone being used to counteract acute rejection.

Antilymphocytic serum

Recently specific antibodies have been raised against lymphocytes, but this has been a costly process and it is the expense and severe anaphylactic reactions and thrombocytopenia that have limited its use. However, short courses have their place and have salvaged many transplants that would otherwise have failed.

Cyclosporin A

This new drug, isolated from fungi, is rapidly becoming the treatment of choice. It is still used with steroids in lower dosage, although recently trials have suggested that it can be used on its own. It is a potent immunosuppressant which may allow less closely matched organs to be used; in fact some units demand only blood group compatibility and have achieved good results.

One of the main problems is nephrotoxicity which occurs when the blood levels rise. Variation in absorption and patient idiosyncrasy are common, and so monitoring of blood levels is an important part of management. Renal damage may be confused with rejection, so the diagnosis has to be confirmed by examination of renal histology of a percutaneous renal biopsy.

Blood transfusions

It has been found empirically that pre-transplant transfusion increases graft survival by an as yet unknown mechanism. Betweeen 1 and 3.5 litres preoperatively seem to be required to provide benefit, although it has been suggested that 200 ml of fresh blood given immediately prior to the transplant provides equally beneficial results. Further studies will be required to place this technique in perspective.

Other measures

Other drugs such as cyclophosphamide, total body and graft irradiation, plasmapheresis and cannulation of the lymphatic duct have all been tried at some stage but are no longer in general use.

Surgical procedure

The majority of kidneys for transplanting are obtained from cadavers and are matched to the most suitable recipient. Permission has to be given by the next of kin and the coroner has to be informed before kidneys are removed.

A relatively small number of kidneys are donated by close relatives, i.e. within siblings and parent to child. Great care is taken to ensure that the donor is willing, that his or her general health is excellent, and that the overall and individual kidney function is normal.

After removal by an experienced surgeon the kidneys are flushed with special solution at 4°C and cooled in ice for transportation.

When a potential donor is being considered, infection, hepatitis, pre-existing renal disease and the presence of a carcinoma are all absolute contraindications, and most units do not accept kidneys from subjects above 65 years old.

The kidney is placed in a retroperitoneal position in the iliac fossa, with a renal artery anastomosed usually end-to-side with the internal iliac artery, while the renal vein is anastomosed in a similar fashion to the external iliac vein. The ureter is implanted through the bladder wall (Fig. 6.2). The recipient may have had recurrent urinary tract infection associated with vesicoureteric reflux, pyelitis and possible hypertension. These are indications for considering pre-transplant nephrectomy. Very large polycystic kidneys may need to be removed, although this is delayed for as long as possible as the functioning renal parenchyma provides erythropoietin, maintaining the haemoglobin at a high level. Patients with abnormal lower urinary tracts require specialist care, and an ileal loop, into which the ureter can be transplanted, may have to be fashioned before the patient is placed on the transplant list.

Postoperative management

Management involves routine care with careful attention to fluid and electrolyte balances.

Following a cadaver graft function may be slow in returning owing to a period of acute tubular necrosis: in that case fluids will need to be restricted and haemodialysis may be required intermittently for 2–3 weeks. In a few cases mannitol and frusemide may promote a diuresis and renal perfusion may be improved with the infusion of dopamine at low doses.

Early function is more frequent following live donor transplantation. In some

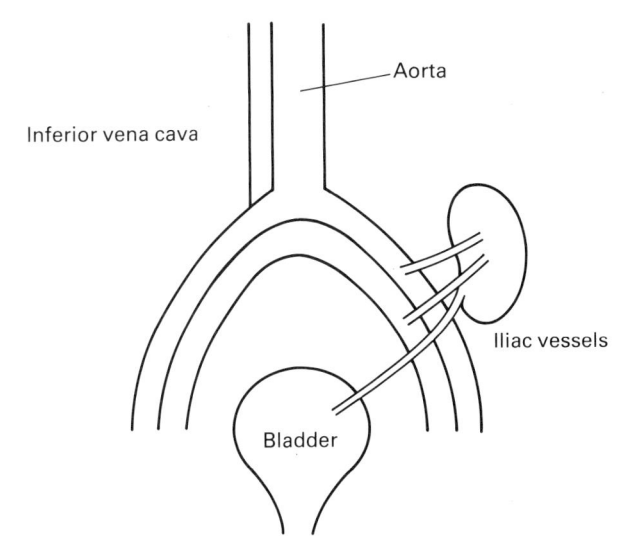

Fig. 6.2 Diagram of the anatomy of a renal transplant.

cases the urine loss may be excessive, requiring careful water, sodium and potassium replacement.

Rejection occurs more frequently during the first 6–8 weeks and is relatively easy to recognize if a graft has already begun to function. However, in the anuric situation it is extremely difficult to make the diagnosis with any certainty.

Recognition of rejection

Hyperacute rejection during the operation results in the kidney becoming cyanosed and flaccid. There is no successful treatment for this.

In contrast, the acute rejection that may occur during the first three months often responds to an increase in steroids given intravenously, or in some cases courses of antilymphocytic globulin. Rejection is not always easy to recognize and during any period of acute reduction in function it has to be distinguished from obstruction, acute tubular necrosis and drug toxicity, in particular due to cyclosporin. The following factors may point towards rejection:

(1) a sudden fall in GFR with a rise in plasma creatinine;
(2) a diminution in urine volume;
(3) an increased temperature;
(4) a feeling of general malaise;
(5) a tender graft – although the graft is denervated, the intense oedema may press on surrounding tissue, causing localized pain;
(6) diminished perfusion and function as detected by the gamma-camera;
(7) an increase in urinary NAG (N-acetylglucosaminidase) – may be a useful indicator but it is not absolute. (There is no specific tubular enzyme that might be liberated by the ischaemia of rejection.)

Ultrasound may demonstrate enlargement of the kidney, and if the calyceal system is enlarged this would support a diagnosis of rejection.

A renal biopsy may be required to distinguish between acute tubular necrosis (ATN), drug toxicity and rejection.

The last two factors assume great importance if the graft has never functioned or if graft function is deteriorating after three months, when the diagnostic possibility begins to favour chronic rejection.

Surgical complications

Of the three anastomoses it is the site of ureteric implantation into the bladder that causes most problems. The blood supply to the lower ureter is carried in the periureteric fat, and if the ureter is too closely dissected during kidney retrieval then ischaemic necrosis with breakdown of the anastomosis produces urinary leakage. Reimplantation or the creation of a funnel of bladder tissue to anastomose directly to the renal pelvis may be required. The use of the patient's own ureter remains an alternative. Apart from urinary leakage, obstruction with impaired graft function may occur and, apart from ischaemia, local oedema and a periureteric haematoma may be responsible.

Leakage from the arterial and venous anastomoses is rare; but a renal artery stenosis may be a late complication, producing hypertension and impaired graft function. Renal vein thrombosis may be a late complication, again associated with poor graft function and often heavy proteinuria.

The large lymphatics of the transplant kidney may be closed by diathermy at the time of operation, but still some patients develop a collection of lymph around the graft – a lymphocoele. A small collection may clear spontaneously and present no problem; but a large collection may compress the ureter, causing obstruction, or may even become infected, producing severe septicaemia. Repeated aspiration under local anaesthesia or continuous drainage may be required. If the lymphocoele persists then surgical drainage to the peritoneal cavity is the definitive approach.

The graft may become swollen and tense during rejection and the capsule may split. This is described as transplant rupture. Some surgeons prefer to divide the capsule at the time of operation to prevent this complication. The splitting may be accompanied by severe bleeding, which unfortunately may lead to removal of the graft.

Medical complications

Acute tubular necrosis may occur in the immediate postoperative period owing to prolonged graft anoxia. Septicaemia developing from whatever cause may also produce a similar end result. The patient needs to be supported by dialysis, and there is usually a satisfactory return in function.

The main medical complications are those associated with immunosuppression. Immediate problems include bone marrow depression and associated sepsis. This may be with an expected bacterial pathogen producing wound, lung and urinary sepsis. More unlikely organisms can be involved, producing the so-called 'opportunist infection'. The following notes outline this clinical problem, which admittedly has become less common with the introduction of cyclosporin and the use of lower levels of steroid.

Viral infections

Cytomegalovirus (CMV) produces a fever, thrombocytopenia and leucopenia, often within 4-10 weeks after transplantation. Joint and muscle pain, and a palpable spleen and liver, complete the picture, while encephalitis is an obvious serious complication. Often a severe pneumonia is a terminal event. The diagnosis is confirmed by an increase in antibody titre and there is no specific treatment. Immunosuppression may need to be discontinued despite the risk of graft failure.

Herpes simplex produces the characteristic labial and oral lesions from which the virus can be isolated. Serious hepatitis, pneumonia and encephalitis may develop. Again a reduction in immunosuppression may be required, while covering the lesions with idoxuridine or using acyclovir may be beneficial. There is only a slight increase in the incidence of chicken-pox, hepatitis B, poliomyelitis and influenza infection.

Opportunist bacterial infections

Listeria monocytogenes produces meningoencephalitis and can easily be cultured from the cerebrospinal fluid. Fortunately, if diagnosed early, the condition responds well to antibiotic therapy.

Nocardia asteroides may produce general malaise, fever, pain and a nodular lesion seen on the chest X-ray. Laboratory isolation is not frequent as the organism is slow-growing and laboratories must be warned, if there is a high index of suspicion, to allow prolonged culture. The organism is sensitive to most antibiotics.

Clostridium difficile can produce a pseudomembranous colitis. The condition may respond to oral vancomycin or metronidazole, and cross-infection should be prevented.

Fungal infections

Aspergillus produces predominantly a pulmonary infection with nodular lesions developing with abscess formation. A good response to amphotericin B can be expected.

Candida often starts as an oral or oesophageal infection but can be widespread, and in severe cases can result in septicaemia. When this occurs the prognosis is poor, despite treatment with amphotericin and 5-fluorocytosine.

Finally, the protozoan infection with *Pneumocystis carinii* may produce pulmonary infection, and here the treatment of choice is cotrimoxazole.

Other complications

Apart from the above complications of infection, steroids may produce glucose intolerance, acute psychosis and may lead to cataract formation and aseptic necrosis of the femoral head. Unfortunately there is also an increased risk of malignancy in the immunosuppressed patient.

Other medical complications include:

(1) acute stress ulceration of the stomach associated with bleeding and perforation;
(2) pulmonary emboli;
(3) nephrotoxicity due to drugs, with particular reference to cyclosporin and the aminoglycosides;
(4) pancreatitis;
(5) a recurrence of glomerulonephritis which may have led to renal failure in the first place. In particular, focal glomerulosclerosis and proliferative lesions are most likely to recur.

There can be no doubt that the quality of life increases enormously with a functioning graft and, unless there are strong contraindications, all patients with renal failure should be considered for renal transplantation. With the use of cyclosporin A, more elderly patients can be treated with fewer postoperative complications, and the two-year graft survival has increased from over 70 per cent to the most recent figure of nearly 90 per cent.

7
Proteinuria and glomerulonephritis

During the process of ultrafiltration in the glomerulus only proteins of a small molecular weight are filtered. The characteristics of the endothelium of the capillary wall, the basement membrane and the epithelial cells of the capsule behave as though they were a semi-permeable membrane with a pore size of approximately 3 nm. Any small-molecular-weight proteins that are filtered are normally reabsorbed by the tubular cells so that only a very small amount of protein (approximately 60 mg) appears in the urine per 24 hours. This figure includes the small amount of the Tamm Horsfall mucoprotein secreted by the tubular cells themselves. Damage to the glomerulus may allow proteins of large molecular weight to be filtered, and if this leak of protein at a glomerular level is considerable then hypoalbuminaemia will develop. When this results in peripheral oedema, the patient is said to have the nephrotic syndrome. Significant proteinuria may be associated with tubular damage, preventing reabsorption of any normally filtered protein, and this tubular proteinuria mainly comprises proteins of low molecular weight (20,000–30,000 daltons). This tubular damage can be associated with many conditions, such as Wilson's disease, the Fanconi syndrome, heavy-metal poisoning and the toxic effects of phenacetin and a persistently low serum potassium.

The causes of a glomerular proteinuria are many; this chapter deals with some, and the reader is also referred to Chapter 15 where the renal involvement in general systemic disease is discussed.

Proteinuria may be discovered as a chance finding during a routine medical examination (e.g. for insurance purposes) or may be detected during the investigation of a patient with a systemic disease. Once detected, the amount of protein excreted in 24 hours should be measured in a timed collection of urine. It should be remembered that a normal increase in proteinuria may be seen after severe exercise or when the patient is in the upright position. The mechanisms of exercise-induced and orthostatic proteinuria are not certain, but they may well be associated with a more sluggish blood flow through the glomeruli owing to vasoconstriction.

Qualitative analysis often provides diagnostic and prognostic information. If only small-molecular-weight proteins are found in the urine, such as albumin (70,000 daltons) and transferrin (90,000 daltons), the proteinuria is said to be *selective*. At the other end of the scale, if large molecules such as IgG (150,000

58 Proteinuria and glomerulonephritis

daltons), fibrin (340,000 daltons) or even the alpha-macroglobulin (820,000 daltons) are passed, then there is considerable damage to the glomerulus and this degree of proteinuria is described as *non-selective*. An index of selectivity can be determined by the IgG/transferrin ratio. An index of 0.2 represents selective proteinuria, while figures of 0.5–0.9 indicate the leakage of predominantly large molecules and is therefore non-selective.

The investigation of the patient with significant proteinuria must include measurement of the glomerular filtration rate, the exclusion of urinary tract infection, and an IVU to exclude major urinary tract abnormalities. The latter is important as quite heavy proteinuria can be associated with urinary tract obstruction.

If this initial screening does not throw light on an obvious cause, then the next step is a renal biopsy. The introduction of the percutaneous renal biopsy in the 1950s has provided valuable information in this group of patients.

Some of the more important causes of proteinuria where the loss is heavy are listed in Table 7.1 (see p. 69). It is clear that a large number of patients will be suffering from an inflammatory process involving the glomeruli, i.e. glomerulonephritis. A detailed analysis is beyond the scope of this chapter. However, as it is a common condition, the student must not only be familiar with the nomenclature of the histological classification, but must also grasp some of the basic immunological principles concerned with pathophysiology and treatment.

Histological classification of glomerulonephritis

A reminder of the organization of the cellular elements within the glomerulus is important at this stage (Hladky and Rink, pp. 48–50). Fig. 7.1 illustrates the organization of the endothelial cells of the capillaries and the epithelial cells. The mesangial cells, which are comparable to the external cells of the normal arteriole, are normally only found at the base or 'stalk' of the numerous capillary loops within the glomerulus. Fig. 7.2 is an electron micrograph of a portion of the basement membrane, and Fig. 7.3 shows a normal glomerulus in a light microscopy section.

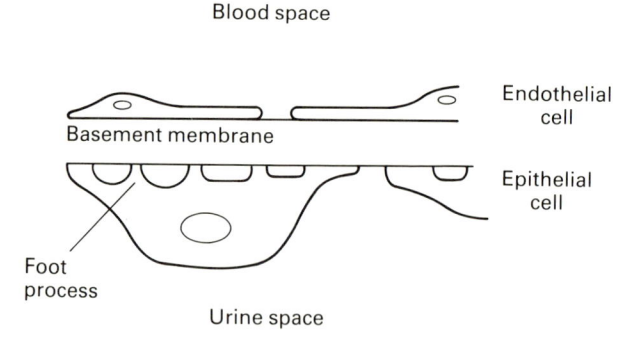

Fig. 7.1 Diagrammatic representation of the organization of the glomerular epithelial and endothelial cells.

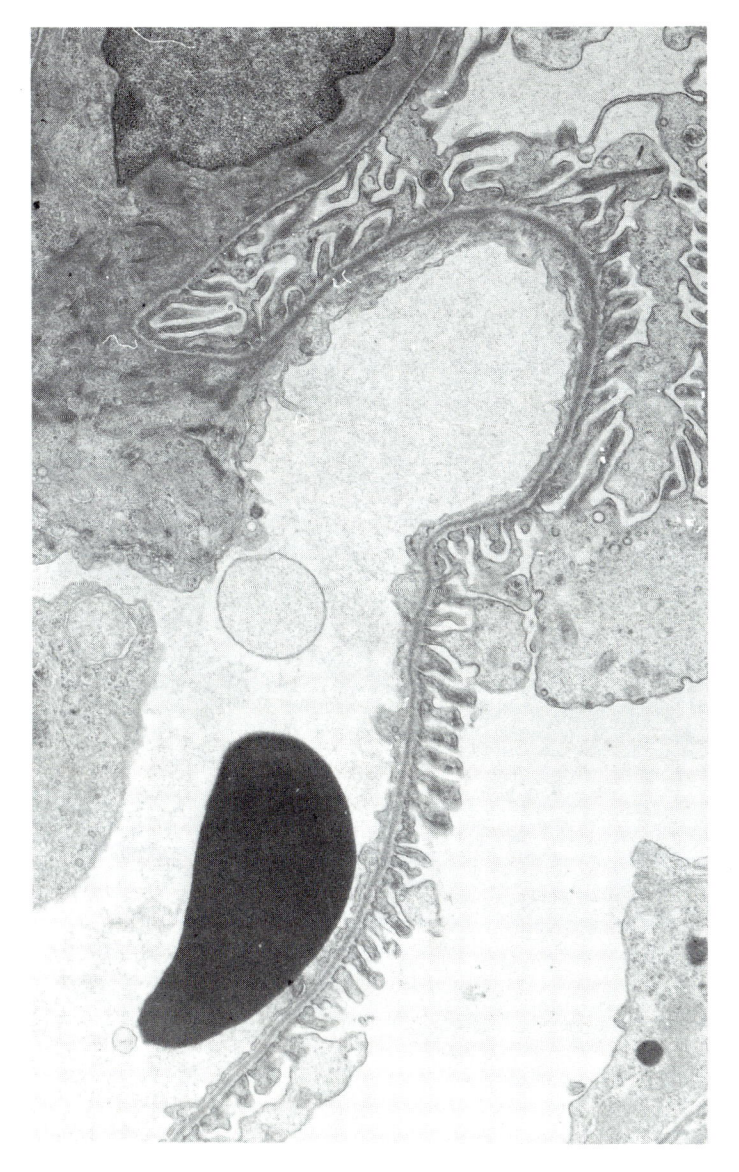

Fig. 7.2 Electron micrograph portion of basement membrane of a normal glomerulus, showing the basement membrane epithelial and endothelial cells (× 13,000).

When describing glomerular involvement the terms used are *diffuse* (all glomeruli involved), *focal* (several involved but some spared), and *segmental* (only part of a glomerulus is damaged).

Examination of sections using the light microscope permits a classification depending on what element of the glomerulus is involved. In practice it may not

60 *Proteinuria and glomerulonephritis*

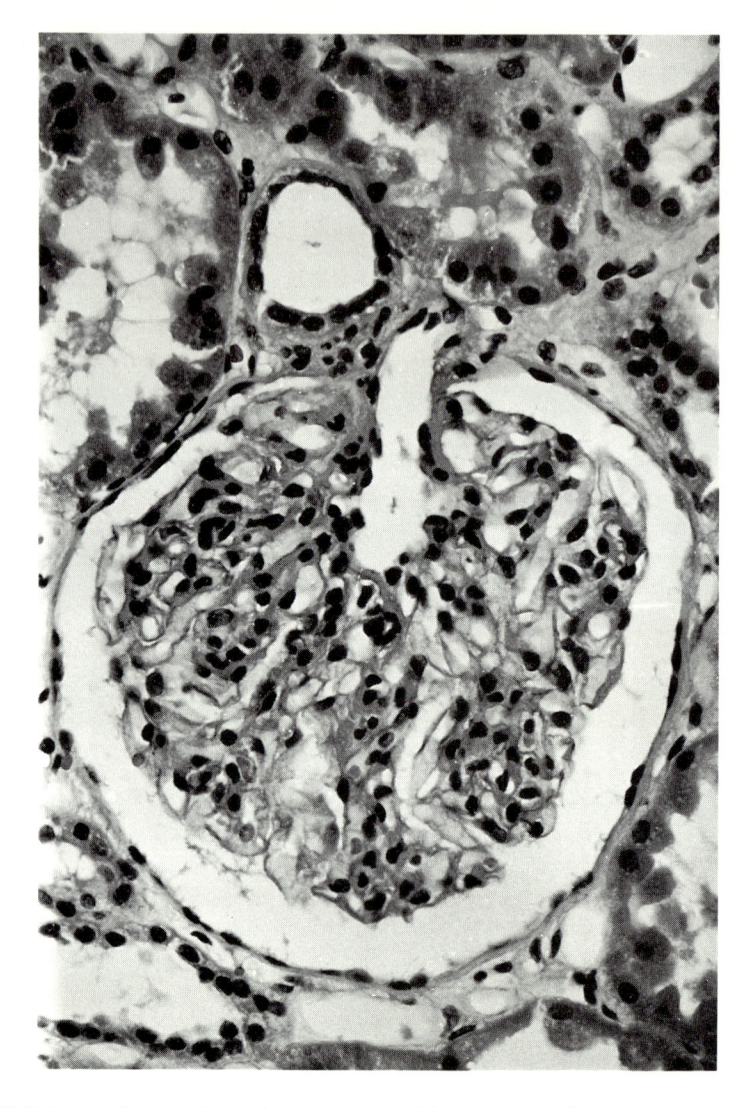

Fig. 7.3 A normal glomerulus as demonstrated by light microscopy, haematoxylin and eosin (× 25 × 20).

be possible to classify the lesion as accurately as the following list would suggest, as a composite picture may be produced with one particular feature dominating. However, some patients do fall into a distinct histological picture and some form of classification is essential to organize this complex pathological situation.

(1) *Minimal-change*: In this condition no obvious gross changes are seen with light microscopy.

(2) *Focal glomerulonephritis*: Small sclerotic areas are seen, commonly close to the juxtaglomerular apparatus.
(3) *Proliferative glomerulonephritis*: We can identify four types:
   (a) *Diffuse* – in this case both the endothelial and mesangial cells have increased in number. The lumina of the capillary tufts are reduced in size by this endothelial proliferation.
   (b) *Mesangial* – the mesangial cells alone are increased in number. The capillary loops are typically patent.
   (c) *Epithelial* – the epithelial cells multiply rapidly and produce crescents that may gradually strangle and obliterate the capillary tufts.
   (d) *Membrano-proliferative* – the proliferation of mesangial cells is associated with thickening of the capillary wall (an alternative name is mesangio-capillary).
(4) *Membranous nephropathy*: Here the basic abnormality is thickening of the capillary walls and basement membrane.

Immunology

The expanding science of immunology is making a valuable contribution to the understanding and treatment of disease. This is quite clearly illustrated in the immunological mechanisms involved in the glomerulonephritic process, both in the experimental animal and man. There are two main ways in which the immune system may damage the glomerulus and cause proteinuria:

(1) by the fixing of circulating immune complexes within the glomerulus; and
(2) by the production of an antibody specifically against the glomerular basement membrane.

Immune complex disease

It is well established that circulating free antibody will combine with circulating antigens to form complexes of varying composition. The immune globulin has two points in the molecule where this union can take place and is therefore described as *divalent*, while antigen may have varying combining sites and can be *monovalent*, *divalent* or *multivalent*. The combination of one molecule of antibody with one of antigen produces a complex that is characteristically non-pathogenic. If the complex contains a predominance of antibody then this complex is removed by the reticuloendothelial system, and it is the complex in which antigen is in excess that is known to cause local tissue damage. This damage is a result of the complex fixing within the tissue and reacting with complement to produce a chain of events that causes platelets and white cells to agglutinate, and mast cells and polymorphs to release vasoactive amines and enzymes to evoke an inflammatory response and alter vascular permeability within the glomerulus.

The conditions for the production of a complex that contains an excess of antigen have to be precise. The readiness of an antigen to combine with an antibody – its *affinity* – must be such that a complex will readily form and the condition of antigen excess must be exact. If a subject is tolerant of a foreign antigen and no antibody is produced, clearly complexes cannot be formed. If the other extreme occurs and there is a brisk and plentiful antibody response, then again insoluble complexes that will be phagocytosed are produced. During the production of antibody there is a period when antigen is in excess and the pathogenic complex is formed. This situation is perpetuated if a low titre of antibody is produced or if the antibody has such a low affinity that it will not readily combine with antigen, and the latter will always remain in excess.

The process can be illustrated in the experimental animal by the production of serum sickness. When bovine albumin is injected into a rabbit the antibody generated forms complexes. As the titre rises there is a stage when antigen is in excess and the complex is deposited in tissue, causing vasculitis, arthralgia, cardiac involvement and a glomerulonephritis. With time, antibody production becomes excessive and the so-called picture of serum sickness ceases.

The use of fluorescent staining techniques has allowed the site of fixation of complexes within the tissues to be visualized histologically. The location either within capillary wall, basement membrane or on the epithelial side of the capillary wall has certain diagnostic features; these will be mentioned when the clinical features are discussed.

Antibodies produced against the basement membrane

This situation can be produced experimentally by injecting antibody raised in another animal against the basement membrane. The clinical counterpart could be when various bacteria or virus particles share a protein almost identical to that found in the basement membrane but sufficiently foreign to raise antibody that combines with and damages the basement membrane. Once the antibody is bound to the basement membrane, the C1q component of complement is activated and this triggers a cascade of events involving platelets and white cell agglutination, and the attraction of polymorphs; these in their turn release lysozymal enzymes that damage the basement membrane and produce inflammation.

In man a rare form of glomerulonephritis is produced when antibodies are generated against the basement membrane. This inappropriate antibody production seems to be associated with infection, and, as the protein of the pulmonary basement membrane is similar, lung damage manifested as haemorrhage also occurs. This antibody can be measured and removed by plasmapheresis. The prognosis of this disease (antiglomerular basement membrane disease – Goodpasture's syndrome) is poor.

Clinical presentation

Glomerulonephritis may present in several ways:

(1) *Acute nephritic syndrome*: There is a reduction in glomerular filtration rate associated with proteinuria, haematuria, oedema and hypertension. Classically seen in patients with poststreptococcal glomerulonephritis, it may produce acute renal failure.

(2) *Asymptomatic proteinuria*: This is often detected during a routine medical examination.
(3) *Asymptomatic haematuria*: There are many causes of haematuria, including trauma, renal calculi, tumour, blood dyscrasias and glomerulonephritis (see Chapter 17). Often when other causes have been excluded, a renal biopsy reveals glomerular damage.
(4) *Nephrotic syndrome*: This is a combination of heavy proteinuria, peripheral oedema, raised cholesterol and lipids.
(5) *Chronic renal failure.*

Common forms of glomerulonephritis

Acute glomerulonephritis

Some patients who develop acute glomerulonephritis have had in the previous month a streptococcal infection. In the early descriptions of the disease this commonly followed scarlet fever, but in recent years episodes of tonsillitis and pharyngitis, and in some cases skin infection with a beta-haemolytic-streptococcus, have been the triggering factors. Not all the streptococci are responsible, and when the published cases are reviewed it appears that groups 12, 4, 1 and 49 are more commonly involved. It is interesting to note that group 12 is not haemolytic and does not produce the streptolysins S and O, and therefore in the clinical course a rise in the ASO titre cannot be expected. Normally this titre rises in about 90 per cent of cases within the first week, reaches a peak 2-3 weeks later and gradually subsides.

The renal damage does not appear to be related directly to the infection *per se*, or to bacterial toxins. The glomerular damage is due to the fixing of soluble immune complexes in the basement membrane, which in turn produces cellular proliferation and damage. When renal biopsy material is examined under the light microscope, all the glomeruli are involved and appear to be hypercellular and swollen. The capillary walls are enlarged and there is both endothelial and mesangial cell proliferation, as well as a large number of polymorphs that have migrated as a result of complement activation. The tubules show relatively little damage, and this lesion fits into the category of a diffuse proliferative glomerulonephritis.

Immunofluorescent staining demonstrates the presence of IgG and C3, which can be seen as a fine, granular luminescence within the capillary walls, and with electron microscopy characteristic humps of electron-dense material are seen on the epithelial surface of the basement membrane. These may well represent immune complexes and they are known to resolve with time. It appears that males are involved more than females and that, although initially it was thought to be primarily a disease of young school-children, there are now almost as many cases reported in the older age groups. Following a latent period of 1-4 weeks after a streptococcal infection, the urine becomes characteristically smoky in appearance owing to free haemoglobin. Microscopy of the urine at this stage demonstrates red cells and red cell and granular casts. The face becomes oedematous, and this may be due to extravasation from damaged capillary walls, although the initial suggestion that the protein content of the oedema fluid was raised has now been discounted. The oedema is more likely to be secondary to the oliguria and severe sodium and water retention that is known to occur. This may also produce hypertension which, though commonly transitory, in rare instances reaches extremely high levels and produces encephalopathy. The bradycardia may be a reflection of direct myocardial involvement.

Routine investigations reveal a reduced glomerular filtration rate and nitrogen retention during the acute phase. Serum complement levels are low, in keeping with the immune background of the disease.

Treatment is mainly symptomatic. The use of penicillin to eradicate the primary infection does not influence the overall prognosis. The outcome in children is good, with only a small percentage dying in the acute phase as a result of cardiac or renal failure. Well over 90 per cent of the children recover without any apparent residual deficit. The outcome in adults is not quite so favourable. Again death can occur in the acute phase, and although the majority recover, 10-15 per cent of patients develop progressive renal failure and either die or would require supportive therapy at the end of the 2-year period.

Rapidly progressive glomerulonephritis

In this heterogeneous group the predominant feature is that the overall prognosis is extremely poor. Renal function deteriorates and supportive haemodialysis is required within weeks or months.

In some cases there is evidence of a preceding streptococcal infection, and in some patients there is no doubt that this represents a rapidly progressive form of the poststreptococcal glomerulonephritic lesion that has been described above. In other instances it is associated with Henoch-Schönlein purpura, polyarteritis nodosa and Goodpasture's syndrome, all of which are discussed in Chapter 15.

Histologically the predominant feature is the proliferation of the capsular epithelium, producing crescents. These crescents can squeeze and ultimately obliterate the glomerular tuft, which is also abnormal owing to proliferation both of mesangial and endothelial cells (Fig. 7.4). The glomerular tuft often demonstrates a lobular appearance and there may be associated areas of scarring. Tubular damage in some instances may be marked. Although the histological picture is not homogeneous, it is quite clearly a proliferative lesion.

This histological picture carries a poor prognosis. Although steroids, cyclophosphamide and azathioprine have been used, recovery is rare, and if patients are to survive they have to be seriously considered for maintenance haemodialysis.

Chronic glomerulonephritis

Many patients who present in middle age with chronic renal failure have a glomerulonephritic lesion. In those patients in whom the glomerular filtration rate is already severely reduced, especially when small kidneys can be demonstrated radiologically, a renal biopsy is often not performed. Examination of

Common forms of glomerulonephritis 65

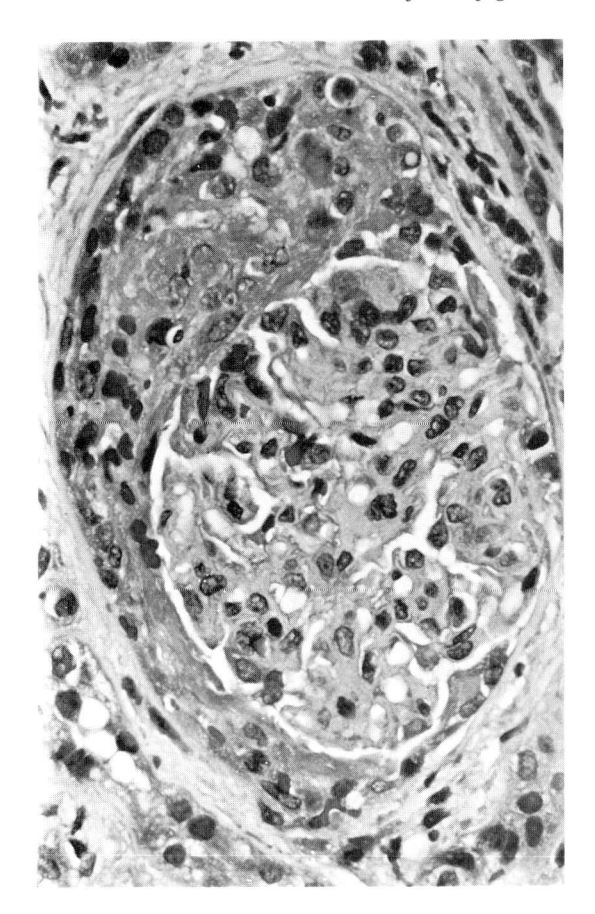

Fig. 7.4 Crescentic glomerulonephritis. Section of glomerulus stained with haematoxylin and eosin, demonstrating proliferative glomerulonephritis with a crescent (top left) (× 25 × 20).

post-mortem material confirms the small kidneys, the capsules of which are closely adherent and do not strip away easily. On the cut surface it is seen that the cortex is thin and pale. Histologically there are no characteristic lesions as the renal failure may have multiple aetiologies. It is often a surprise that some of the glomeruli are completely normal while others are solid owing to the presence of collagen within the Bowman's capsule. This may be the result of crescents becoming organized, or ischaemia. In some instances the appearances of a membranous or membrano-proliferative lesion can be defined. Many of the tubules are lost and those that remain are often atrophic. Some, however, appear dilated, a possible sequela of either obstruction or a compensatory mechanism.

Membranous glomerulonephritis

In this group of patients all the glomeruli are seen to be involved when examined under the light microscope. The capillary walls are thickened and there is no obvious increase in the cellular content of the glomerulus (Fig. 7.5). Initially the capillary lumen is patent, but as the disease advances obliteration is common. This obliteration is due to the deposition of an eosinophilic material that is deposited on the basement membrane. Electron microscopy provides additional information as to the nature of this thickening as, in the early stages, it appears to be due to deposits on the epithelial side of the membrane through which the basement membrane protrudes, giving it a spiky pattern, clearly seen with light microscopy when silver stains are used. The foot processes of the epithelial cells are fused, and with time there appears to be further deposition within the basement membrane, which is grossly thickened, and it is this that ultimately occludes the capillary lumen. Once again, immune complexes appear to be involved in the pathogenesis, since fluorescent staining using antisera against IgG shows a granular deposition within the capillary wall. The fluorescence is not so strong when antisera against C3, IgA and IgM are used. A similar histological picture is seen when chronic serum sickness is produced in the experimental animal.

Clinically these patients present with peripheral oedema and a heavy proteinuria, which may constitute the nephrotic syndrome. Microscopic haematuria is common and on occasion it reaches macroscopic proportions. The proteinuria can be heavy, with 10–15 g being passed per 24 hours, and it is characteristically non-selective. The glomerular filtration rate, if not reduced initially, often shows a steady, downhill trend with the patient reaching end-

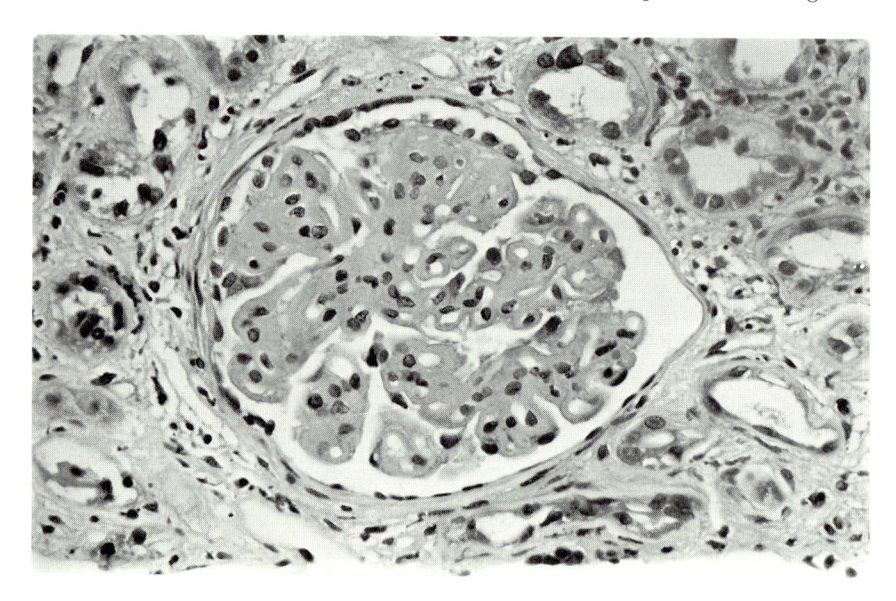

Fig. 7.5 Membranous glomerulonephritis. Section of glomerulus stained with haematoxylin and eosin, demonstrating obvious thickening of the basement membrane (× 25 × 20).

stage renal failure in two or three years. In some cases, however, there is spontaneous remission, but characteristically there is a poor response to steroid therapy.

Membrano-proliferative glomerulonephritis

This is yet another glomerulonephritic process that tends to carry a poor prognosis. Light microscopy shows that all the glomeruli are involved and are much increased in size. Characteristically the capillary tufts have an accentuated lobular pattern and there is patchy thickening of the capillary wall which, on silver staining, may be associated with splitting of the basement membrane. There is a marked increase of mesangial cells, and on occasions epithelial crescents can be seen. Once more, immune complex deposition may be responsible as characteristically there is strong granular fluorescence in the capillary walls against C3. Other immunoglobulins and complement fractions can also be demonstrated.

Characteristically it appears to be a disease of children, although it can present at any stage in life. Presentation can take many forms. It may present as chance proteinuria at a routine medical examination; or, at the other end of the scale, the patient may be nephrotic with heavy, non-selective proteinuria. In some instances the features of acute glomerulonephritis are present, and on occasion the presentation is one of macroscopic haematuria.

Renal function slowly deteriorates, but it may be many years before severe renal functional impairment has occurred. The response to therapy is poor, although there are reports of improvement in function and histology when combination therapy is used. This includes steroids, azathioprine, cyclophosphamide, anticoagulants and antiplatelet therapy in the form of dipyrimadole.

Focal glomerulonephritis

As the description implies, only certain glomeruli are involved, the rest being completely normal. The affected glomeruli may have an area of proliferation at their edge, and in some cases this may involve crescent formation. In another group the focal lesion is primarily due to necrosis owing to small vessel involvement, as is seen in microscopic polyarteritis nodosa. Clinically this type of lesion can be seen in Henoch–Schönlein purpura and systemic lupus erythematosus (see Chapter 15).

A focal lesion may present clinically as chance proteinuria or, if heavy, the nephrotic syndrome. The overall prognosis varies as some patients do surprisingly well, with or without steroid therapy, and in others renal function slowly deteriorates. Of particular interest are those patients who present with recurrent haematuria. The haematuria is macroscopic and is often associated with an upper respiratory tract infection, exercise or prophylactic innoculation. There is no latent period as is seen in poststreptococcal glomerulonephritis – the haematuria being coincidental with the infection or exercise.

The immunofluorescence seen in this lesion is interesting as all the glomeruli fluoresce, despite the lesion being focal. A distinct sub-group appears to be emerging as some patients fluoresce specifically with antisera against IgA.

Minimal-change nephritis

As the descriptive title suggests there are often no changes to be detected with light microscopy. The pathological features, however, are seen with electron microscopy. Typically there is fusion of the foot processes of the epithelial cells. During periods of remission it is clear that these foot processes reform in their normal configuration. There is no typical pattern with immunofluorescence, although certain cases illustrate deposits of IgE.

An alternative title for this condition is 'lipoid nephrosis'. This descriptive title arose from the fact that in the urine of patients numerous fat bodies can be seen. Clinically this presents typically as the nephrotic syndrome in young children: by and large there is a good response to steroids and it appears that the natural history of the disease is one of remission. When presenting in adult life the overall prognosis is good, especially as again there is a prompt reduction in proteinuria with steroid therapy.

Nephrotic syndrome

It is appropriate to discuss the nephrotic syndrome at the end of this chapter since it is often due to glomerulonephritis.

The major feature of this syndrome is heavy proteinuria, which in turn leads to a low serum albumen. When the albumen concentration falls below 1.6 g%, then the colloid osmotic pressure is insufficient to hold fluid within the vascular compartment and there is a leakage into the interstitial space, with a secondary fall in the circulating plasma volume. This reduced plasma volume leads to sodium and water retention by the kidney. This is mediated first by a reduction in the glomerular filtration rate, and second via aldosterone. Quite independent of these mechanisms there is often an associated hypercholesterolaemia and an alteration in the lipid profile.

Table 7.1 lists the more common causes of the nephrotic syndrome.

Aetiological factors

Since the glomerulonephritic process has already been covered in detail, some of the more important remaining aetiological factors will be commented on briefly.

Renal vein thrombosis

A rise in the venous pressure is often associated with proteinuria. The underlying mechanisms are not certain because examination of renal biopsy material reveals no pathognomonic changes. The glomeruli are by and large normal, and the bulk of the pathology seems to lie in the tubules which are dilated and have flattened epithelia. There is often interstitial oedema leading to separation of the tubules.

A significant rise in venous pressure producing proteinuria may be associated with congestive cardiac failure, constrictive pericarditis and tricuspid valve disease. However, apart from these cardiac problems, thrombosis of the inferior

Nephrotic syndrome 69

Table 7.1 Common causes of heavy proteinuria and the nephrotic syndrome

Glomerulonephritis as a primary renal disorder
  Minimal-change
  Membranous
  Proliferative
Glomerulonephritis associated with general disease
  Bacterial endocarditis
  Syphilis
  Malaria
  Systemic lupus erythematosus
  Polyarteritis
  Malignancy
  Henoch–Schönlein purpura
Amyloid
Diabetes
Renal transplant
Pre-eclampsia of pregnancy
Drugs (e.g. gold, tolbutamide, penicillamine)
Allergic (e.g. bee stings)
Cardiovascular
  Renal vein thrombosis
  Constrictive pericarditis

vena cava or the renal veins themselves can produce heavy proteinuria. As far as renal vein thrombosis is concerned, the patient may complain of spontaneous lumbar pain associated with haematuria and a picture of acute renal failure may develop. There is a high incidence of renal vein thrombosis being associated with amyloidosis. It is difficult to be certain about the prognosis since often, with or without the use of anticoagulants, the veins recanalize and renal function returns to a degree that can support normal life. However, a certain number of patients perish in acute renal failure.

Drugs

When mercurial diuretics were used extensively to treat congestive cardiac failure, a small proportion of patients developed the nephrotic syndrome. The industrial use of mercury has also been blamed, and necrosis of the proximal convoluted tubule appears to be the major pathological feature.

The gold salts used by rheumatologists can also produce heavy proteinuria. In these cases, as well as tubular damage, there is thickening of the basement membrane associated with the deposition of electron-dense deposits when viewed with the electron microscope. A similar pattern can also be seen when penicillamine is used to treat patients with cystinuria.

Syphilis

In the congenital form of syphilis there is evidence of deposition of immune complexes that fluoresce with IgM and IgG in the subepithelial region of the basement membrane. There is a more cellular response in the glomeruli in cases of secondary syphilis. The response to penicillin treatment in both instances is usually good.

Malaria

Infection with *Plasmodium malariae* can produce the nephrotic syndrome. It is clearly an immune complex disease. In some patients the glomerular lesion is predominantly proliferative, while in others the brunt of the damage seems to be borne by the basement membrane.

Malignant disease

The nephrotic syndrome is a rare but interesting manifestation of malignant disease. It is clearly an immune complex phenomenon in which antibodies are made against the neoplasm, and the resultant complexes fix within the glomeruli.

Specific clinical problems

There are specific problems common to all patients with nephrotic syndrome.

Owing to the excessive protein loss there may be a poor nutritional state, with osteoporosis, striae of the skin, muscle wasting and hair loss. Obviously if the underlying lesion can be corrected that is ideal, but a high-protein diet may help to combat the urinary wastage. Occasionally in severe cases hypovolaemia develops, and intravenous replacement of protein may be required since severe hypotension may lead on to poor renal perfusion and acute renal failure.

Oedema can be severe and may require, again, intravenous protein administration, oral sodium restriction and the use of diuretics. Clearly protein replacement is just a temporary measure until an attempt can be made at more definitive treatment.

Owing to the low levels of gammaglobulin, infections are a problem and appropriate antibiotics are required.

Thrombosis, possibly associated with haemoconcentration and increased fibrinogen levels, can be a clinical problem. Periods of immobilization should be avoided. Once a thrombosis has developed, anticoagulation should be commenced.

There is an increased risk of myocardial infarction, possibly precipitated by low blood pressure and hypovolaemia, with the raised plasma lipids producing coronary artery disease.

8

Systemic hypertension

Arterial hypertension is a common, life-threatening disease that can affect all age groups. A raised pressure, however produced, damages the arterioles. If the pressure rise is rapid and severe, as in accelerated or 'malignant' hypertension, then fibrin is produced within the vessel wall, and this pink, eosinophilic material can rapidly occlude the lumen, producing distal ischaemia.

A modest pressure rise that develops gradually over several years narrows the calibre of the vessels, not by fibrinoid necrosis but by a reduplication of the internal elastic lamina and increased cellularity of the vessel wall. These changes are difficult to reverse, with the possible exception of the fibrinoid change associated with severe hypertension for which prompt, effective treatment may produce a surprising degree of resolution.

In contrast, the hypertrophy of benign hypertension is permanent, and so clearly 'prevention is better than cure'. Clinically this is now possible as modern treatment is both better tolerated by the patient and more effective. Gone are the days of severe postural hypotension, certain impotence, sedation, etc., associated with early ganglion blocking drugs used twenty-five years ago. With the advent of beta-adrenergic blockade and peripheral dilators, modern therapy, which is relatively free of problems, allows more patients to be treated for milder forms of hypertension; thus the physician hopes to prevent severe organ damage. The arteriolar narrowing affects mainly the heart, kidney and fundus of the eye, with cerebral and intestinal vessels being involved less frequently.

The systemic circulation is represented by a pump (the left ventricle) and a series of pipes (the arterial tree). Poiseuille, a French physicist and physiologist, defined the relationship between pressure and flow in a rigid pipe:

$$Q = \Delta P \times \frac{\pi r^4}{8L} \times \frac{1}{\rho}$$

where Q is the volume per unit time, ΔP is the pressure gradient along the vessel, r is the radius, L is the length, and ρ is the coefficient of viscosity. From this it is clear that the central factor governing the pressure is the diameter of the pipe, and small changes in the radius result in major pressure changes. This explains why small fluctuations in arteriolar tone produce major fluctuations in pressure.

It is at the arteriolar level that the major pressure drop occurs, and the degree of constriction is largely dependent on the sympathetic tone influencing the α-adrenoreceptors. These vessels produce the major resistance to flow – the peripheral resistance – which in the majority of hypertensive patients is raised. In the accelerated form the resistance is very high and is the major circulatory abnormality, while in other hypertensive patients variations in pump activity – the cardiac output – may also play a part. The relationship between the cardiac output and resistance to flow is as follows:

blood pressure
= cardic output × peripheral resistance × viscosity

Variations in blood viscosity appear to play little part in the clinical management of patients. In some patients the blood pressure is labile, fluctuating from hour to hour, and in this group the cardiac output is usually elevated, possibly associated with periods of stress. There is evidence to suggest that a raised cardiac output may lead to hypertension which in time is sustained by a rise in the peripheral resistance, with the cardiac output falling to normal values.

The levels of cardiac output and peripheral resistance vary enormously in the hypertensive population. At one end of the scale the cardiac output may be high, as in the labile group, with the peripheral resistance being only moderately elevated; in the other group with accelerated, severe hypertension the cardiac output may even be below normal, with the pressure being maintained by an extremely high peripheral resistance. Many techniques can be used clinically to measure the cardiac output, but the peripheral resistance is a figure calculated from the cardiac output and the mean blood pressure.

The clinical assessment of the hypertensive patient must answer three main questions:

(1) What is the aetiology of the hypertension, and in particular is there a lesion that can be corrected surgically?
(2) What end-organ damage has there been (particularly to the heart, kidney and eyes)?
(3) What, in the light of the aetiology, is the most appropriate form of treatment?

Aetiology

The role of the kidneys in the production or maintenance of a raised systemic pressure is discussed in Chapter 15 of Hladky and Rink. Our understanding of the pathophysiological mechanisms that produce a raised systemic pressure is far from complete. In cases of phaeochromocytoma, a catecholamine-producing tumour, hyperaldosteronism, and coarctation of the aorta, the sequence of events is fairly clear (see *Clinical Endocrinology* by P. Daggett, in the Physiological Principles in Medicine Series). However, as far as the kidney is concerned the mechanisms involved are not clear, and hence clinical management is not always straightforward. Early clinicians reported the association between renal disease and hypertension, and it is this relationship between the kidney and a raised pressure that needs to be considered and an attempt made to relate the often complex pathophysiology to clinical management.

The renal artery occlusion experiments of Goldblatt in the 1930s produced convincing evidence that renal ischaemia produces a pressure rise, and so considerable attention has been paid to a search for renal artery stenosis. It is also clear that the kidney produces vasodilator substances – kinins and prostaglandins – a lack of which allows vasoconstriction and hypertension to develop; this is so-called 'renoprival hypertension'. A detailed account of these topics cannot be provided here but the student requires an outline to gain a perspective for patient management.

Renal artery stenosis

Occlusion of a renal artery is usually due to extensive atheroma, but in young females thickening of the muscular coat – fibromuscular hypoplasia – may be present. Significant renal arterial narrowing may only account for 5 per cent of the adult hypertensive population, while renovascular problems may be the causative factor in 25 per cent of childhood cases.

As has already been stated, the exact mechanisms are not clear. Certain salient facts are, however, appropriate to clinical management. When renal perfusion is reduced owing to a stenotic lesion of the major renal artery, the renal perfusion pressure is reduced and the kidney is relatively anoxic, and these two factors (amongst others) promote renin release with the increased production of angiotensin II (Fig. 8.1). This results in intense vasoconstriction, stimulation of antidiuretic hormone release, and an increased production of adrenaline and noradrenaline by the suprarenal medulla. Aldosterone is also produced, leading to sodium and water retention. The ischaemic kidney retains sodium and water and the urine flow is reduced.

If the opposite kidney is absent, then this sodium and water retention leads to expansion of the circulating volume which, by an as yet unknown mechanism, dampens down renin release. Peripheral renin activity returns towards

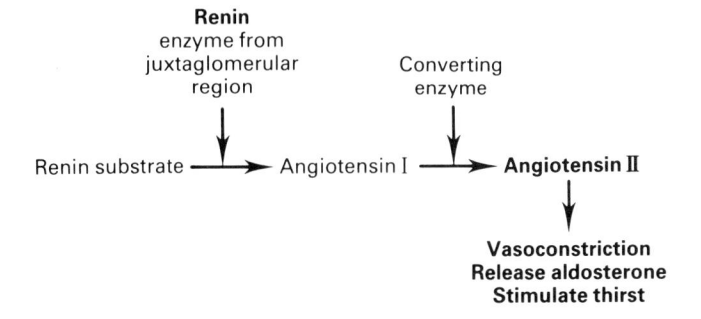

Fig. 8.1 Diagrammatic representation of the renin–angiotensin system.

74 *Systemic hypertension*

normality, and the hypertension is maintained by an expansion of the circulating volume and a rise in the peripheral resistance. If the opposite kidney is present and normal, the increased systemic pressure produces a natriuresis, balancing the sodium retention produced by the ischaemic kidney. The circulatory volume remains normal and the hypertension is driven by increased renin production. With time, however, if the blood pressure is untreated, it damages the renal vessels of the opposite and originally normal kidney and the ability to excrete high levels of sodium is lost, the circulatory volume increases, and once again renin production falls; now the blood pressure is maintained by an expanded circulatory volume and its associated rise in peripheral resistance.

Several reasons for the increase in peripheral resistance have been put forward:

(1) The increased circulating volume produces a rise in the cardiac output, which leads to an increased tissue perfusion; and it is this increased peripheral blood flow that produces a rise in the peripheral resistance. The increased tone of the arterioles may be mediated by an as yet unidentified hormone that interferes with sodium and potassium transport across the cell membrane.
(2) There is evidence that the sympathetic tone is increased and that the vessels have an increased sensitivity to normal circulating levels of catecholamines.
(3) There is evidence to suggest that there is a decreased level of circulating vasodilator substances such as the bradykinins and prostaglandins.

Clearly renal artery stenosis must be excluded in patients with severe hypertension, especially in the younger age groups. As will be seen later, some patients respond to surgical correction of the lesion, thus avoiding life-long oral medication. A vascular bruit may be present, the kidney radiologically may be smaller and, because of the selective sodium and water retention, the nephrogram phase of an IVU will be delayed and appear of greater density. The pyelogram phase will also appear denser on the stenotic side. Renal scintigraphy will confirm the impaired perfusion, and the peak activity recorded on a probe renogram will also be reduced in amplitude and delayed. During a water provoked diuresis the peak on the normal side will occur sooner, but the peak activity from the stenotic side will remain relatively fixed in time and amplitude (Fig. 8.2). Aortography may produce the definitive diagnosis, but the severity of the stenosis from a single plain view is difficult to assess. The use of venous injection of contrast with background subtraction allows visualization of the arterial tree. This technique, which avoids arterial catheterization and the associated risk of dislodging atheromatous plaques, is a recent advance that helps in the diagnosis of this condition.

Choice of treatment

Not all patients become normotensive if the lesion is corrected surgically by end-arterectomy or bypass procedures. Is it possible, therefore, to predict a successful outcome to surgery?

Measurement of the peripheral and renal vein plasma renin activity are

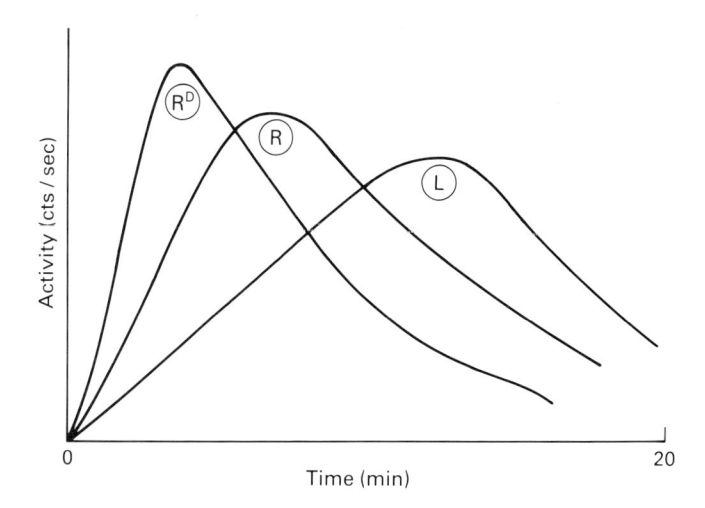

Fig. 8.2 Probe renograms of renal artery stenosis in the oliguric and diuretic phase, demonstrating the delayed and fixed peak resulting from left renal artery stenosis. Following a fluid load the right kidney responds by producing an earlier peak (R^D), while the curve from the left renal region stays relatively unchanged.

helpful, especially if the ratio of renal vein renin activity is above 1.5:1.0 comparing the stenotic with the normal contralateral kidney. Initially high hopes were held for the response to inhibition of the renin–angiotensin system. Saralasin, a synthetic compound capable of selectively blocking the effect of angiotensin II, has been used as a preoperative assessment. If the blood pressure fell significantly following the infusion of saralasin then it was hoped that long-term benefit would be gained by surgery. Unfortunately a reduction in pressure with the infusion does not guarantee long-term benefits from surgery. Blocking the effect of the converting enzyme using oral captopril, thereby limiting the production of angiotensin II, has also been tried, but again its predictive value is not absolute.

The pathophysiology of hypertension associated with renal artery stenosis is complex and it is not easy to predict those patients who will benefit from surgery. However, it may be that the use of balloon catheters to dilate the stenotic lesion may do away with the need for invasive and dangerous surgery. The catheter inserted into the arterial system can be used to inject contrast media and confirm the diagnosis, and the balloon can be inflated across the stenosis, thereby increasing renal blood flow. Percutaneous angioplasty is a relatively non-invasive technique and can be repeated after several weeks if the blood pressure has not fallen to satisfactory levels. At best this relatively simple technique may do away with open surgery by abolishing the high blood pressure completely. In those patients in whom a complete cure has not been achieved it may well reduce the dose of oral medication required. Such a non-invasive procedure is to be welcomed. Further studies are required to assess its value, but if it prevents dangerous surgery in patients who have renal atheroma as part of a widespread disease involving possibly the coronary vessels, then the peroperative risk of cardiac arrhythmias, ischaemia and even cardiac infarction are reduced by avoiding major surgery.

Hypertension associated with renal disease apart from renal artery stenosis

Chronic renal failure

As the glomerular filtration rate diminishes to single figures, sodium and water retention occur. This leads to expansion of the circulating blood volume and an elevation of the blood pressure. In some patients the blood pressure will return to normal once dialysis has been commenced, reducing the blood volume towards normality; but in at least 50 per cent of patients, despite reduction in body weight, the blood pressure remains elevated and it is clear that additional mechanisms are responsible. It is certain that in some patients there is a paradoxical increase in renin production despite an expanded circulation.

Renoprival hypertension

Any pathological process that results in loss of renal parenchyma may be associated with hypertension. This can in part be due to the lack of vasodilator substances that are normally produced by the healthy kidney, including prostaglandins and kinins.

Urinary tract obstruction

If this is associated with severe renal failure then sodium retention may be a factor. However, there is evidence from experimental studies that – certainly early on in the course of obstruction – the plasma renin activity is increased.

Renin secreting tumours

These are very rare. The tumours are rich in secretory granules capable of releasing renin. Surgical removal is invariably effective.

Non-renal causes of hypertension

For the sake of completeness it is important to mention non-renal causes of hypertension. It is important in any patient assessment to exclude these additional factors.

Phaeochromocytoma

This is a tumour of chromaffin tissue mainly found in the suprarenal glands but also sometimes in the mediastinum, para-aortic glands or even the bladder.

A history of paroxysmal tachycardia, headaches and skin pallor is suggestive. The diagnosis is confirmed by measurements of noradrenaline and adrenaline and their breakdown products in urine and plasma.

Localization is now much safer with computer assisted tomography and ultrasound. Surgical removal with careful preoperative preparation is often successful, but long-term follow-up is essential as a small number are malignant and re-occur (see *Clinical Endocrinology* by P. Daggett).

Conn's syndrome

This condition is caused by either a discrete tumour or hyperplasia of the adrenal cortex.

The classical findings of hypokalaemia associated with alkalosis are suggestive in the absence of diuretic therapy. Aldosterone measurements confirm the diagnosis, and the tumour may be identified by ultrasound. (Many elderly patients have benign adrenal adenomas, and so the presence of a tumour and hypertension is not adequate proof in these cases.) Surgery is normally required.

It is interesting that the hypertension is associated with a high circulating blood volume and cardiac output, with only modest elevation in the peripheral resistance (see *Clinical Endocrinology* by P. Daggett).

Coarctation of the aorta

Narrowing of the aorta at the level of the insertion of the ductus arteriosus may produce hypertension in the upper limbs. Collaterals develop, and the increased flow through the internal mammary vessels often erodes the posterior aspects of the ribs, producing the classical rib notching seen on a chest X-ray. Surgery is indicated.

Essential hypertension

Despite the screening of hypertensive patients for the above surgically correctable lesions, in the majority of patients no such lesion is found and the label of 'essential hypertension' is given.

For many years a pathophysiological mechanism for this large group has been sought. There is some evidence to suggest that there may be a renal abnormality that produces abnormal sodium and water homeostasis with inappropriate sodium retention, leading to an expansion of the circulating blood volume. In response to increased tissue perfusion, there is an autoregulatory mechanism leading to an increased peripheral resistance.

Excess production of noradrenaline has been suggested. It is difficult to demonstrate elevated circulating levels, but certainly there is a suggestion that the arterioles may over-respond to normal circulating levels, producing inappropriate vasoconstriction.

Assessment of end-organ damage

The kidneys

The glomerular arterioles and capillaries can be occluded both by fibrinoid and by hyaline degeneration, leading to a gradual diminution in the glomerular filtration rate.

The deterioration in function may be rapid in those patients in whom the blood pressure rises quickly and to a high level, whereas the majority of patients with a more modest rise in pressure present for many years may show only a gradual reduction in function.

Routine measurements of plasma creatinine and creatinine clearance are essential, not only as a baseline assessment but also to follow progress: with the reduction in pressure by medical treatment, renal perfusion will be reduced and, as the normal intrarenal autoregulation of blood flow is impaired, this may lead to a further reduction in the glomerular filtration rate.

This reduction in function has to be accepted, but there is evidence that some drugs may produce an inappropriate loss in function. In particular the beta-adrenergic blocking drugs have been blamed for precipitating renal failure in a small group of patients. The evidence is not striking; but when the converting enzyme inhibitors such as captopril are used they may indeed produce marked reduction in function in those patients who have a renal artery stenosis. Here the perfusion of glomeruli is dependent on high renin and angiotensin II levels, and a reduction in these levels due to converting enzyme inhibition may lead to a dramatic fall in function. This is thought to be due to a reduction in glomerular filtration pressure as a result of dilatation of the efferent arteriole. The same sequence of events has been described in patients without proven renal artery stenosis, and it is postulated that it is the smaller interlobular vessels that are narrowed leading to activation of the renin–angiotensin system. Fortunately, stopping the drug is usually associated with a return in function.

The heart

Sustained, elevated systemic pressure will place an increased workload on the left ventricle, leading to hypertrophy and strain. A history of dyspnoea or chest pain is important as there may be pre-existing coronary artery disease or the severe muscle hypertrophy may produce relative ischaemia.

Whatever the mechanism, it is clear that the anaemia of renal failure will embarrass cardiac performance even further. In addition to the clinical examination a chest X-ray may reveal cardiac enlargement with or without pulmonary oedema, while the ECG may illustrate left ventricular enlargement and/or ischaemia.

The eyes

In cases of accelerated hypertension, visual impairment may be severe owing to retinal haemorrhages, especially in the area of the macula. Successsful treatment may produce slow resolution and improvement in vision, but unfortunately some patients may be left with permanent disability. Other ophthalmic findings include exudates and papilloedema, and thickening of the vessels in the more benign forms.

Treatments

If there is evidence of severe end-organ damage, then the patient should be regarded as a medical emergency and every effort should be made to reduce the diastolic pressure to 90 mmHg or below.

Modern hypotensive agents act within hours, and the need to reduce the pressure rapidly with intravenous medication is rare. Severe pulmonary oedema caused by hypertension is perhaps the only clinical indication for rapid pressure reduction. With the introduction of the beta-adrenergic blocking drugs in the late 1970s patient management has become easier now that the ganglion blocking drugs are no longer used.

A detailed pharmacological review will not be given and the student must refer to a standard text for precise details of dosage and side-effects. However, the salient points will be presented, with particular reference to renal function.

Diuretics

The thiazide group are traditionally the first line of treatment for mild to moderate hypertension in those patients with no organ damage. These agents appear to exert their acute effect by reducing the circulating volume and lowering the body's exchangeable sodium. They also act directly on the vessel wall, producing vasodilatation. Patients sometimes complain of the inconvenience of an abrupt diuresis, and the longer acting agents such as chlorthalidone are equally effective and better tolerated.

Any diuretic may be used but they are not without problems. Uric acid retention and gout, glucose intolerance, impotence and postural hypotension are among the common complaints. The theoretical disadvantage of causing hypovolaemia, which stimulates the renin–angiotensin system, must not be overlooked.

Beta-adrenergic blockade

With the introduction of propranolol a new era of hypotensive treatment began. The mode of action of this group of drugs is not clear. A reduction in cardiac output is certainly not the sole factor, but in those patients with a labile blood pressure and a high resting cardiac output, often associated with stress, clearly a reduction in cardiac output is important. The speed of ejection from the left ventricle is reduced and the rate of pressure rise across the baroreceptors is also diminished, and this may be an important factor in the so-called 'resetting' of the baroreceptors, lowering their threshold of stimulation and thereby reducing the sympathetic tone.

Fat-soluble compounds such as propanolol pass the blood–brain barrier easily and may exert a central effect on the cerebral cortex. Renin production is partly under the control of the sympathetic nervous system and reduced renin production may be another hypotensive mechanism.

Dosage is important. Some clinicians feel that very high doses can be used with benefit, but this is debatable.

A second generation of drugs was developed which block the beta-receptors

80 Systemic hypertension

in the heart, leaving the peripheral and pulmonary receptors relatively untouched, thereby reducing the risk of bronchospasm and cold extremities which are common complaints with these agents. The so-called 'selective' drugs, of which atenolol is an example, are now becoming the drugs of choice.

A past history of bronchospasm and cardiac failure mean that this approach cannot be used unless the patient is carefully monitored in hospital. The biological half-life of these drugs is long and daily administration is often efficient, a factor in favour of better patient compliance.

A fall in pressure may occur within 12–24 hours of oral administration. If a more rapid response is required then vasodilating agents may be given simultaneously.

Vasodilators

Agents such as hydralazine which act directly on the blood vessel wall are potent hypotensive agents. However, with the fall in blood pressure the sympathetic system is stimulated in an attempt to maintain the status quo, and the resultant reflex tachycardia produces palpitations and often angina. For these reasons their use alone has been discontinued.

With the advent of beta-adrenergic blockade this secondary response has been blunted, and combination therapy has been introduced with benefit. There is a suggestion that when the two agents are used together the vasodilator may maintain renal function by increasing renal blood flow.

Hydralazine can be given intramuscularly or intravenously in cases of emergency if the oral route is inappropriate. Joint pain and a lupus-like syndrome can occur when hydralazine is given in doses above 200 mg daily. Other dilating agents such as sodium nitroprusside can only be given intravenously (and are often only for emergency use), while other compounds such as diazoxide and minoxidil can be given orally. Excessive hair growth and sodium and water retention leading to oedema often limit the use of minoxidil, although the latter can be overcome with simultaneous diuretic administration.

Alpha-adrenergic blocking agents

Vasoconstrictor tone is mediated by the alpha-adrenergic receptor. Blocking agents have been tried with little success, as the response is short-lived with the vessels becoming rapidly refractory.

Labetalol possesses both alpha- and beta-adrenergic blocking properties, and when given intravenously it produces an immediate fall in pressure without a rise in pulse rate. For this reason it is a useful drug in the management of phaeochromocytoma and hypertensive crisis in the severely ill patient. When labetalol is given orally the pressure falls within 4 hours owing to the alpha-blocking component, and it is a useful drug for long-term use.

Prazosin has alpha-adrenergic blocking properties, although it was originally classified primarily as a vasodilator acting directly on smooth muscle. Postural hypotension is a problem, mainly when the first dose is given or if high doses are used.

Converting enzyme inhibitors

The most widely used agent of this group, which prevents the production of angiotensin II, is captopril. In those patients whose hypertension is clearly maintained by a high renin production, the drug should be used cautiously as severe hypotension may occur. This compound may also produce the nephrotic syndrome, neuropathy and marrow depression, and it should therefore be reserved for severe refractory hypertension.

Calcium antagonists

These are a new group of compounds of which nifedipine is now widely used. These compounds cause peripheral vasodilatation, partly by their effect on calcium ion movement in smooth muscle. They also have a negative inotropic effect on the heart and have been used for angina and arrhythmias. For this reason they are useful in those patients who have cardiac problems associated with their hypertension.

9

Infections of the urinary tract

Cystitis

Patients have various ideas of the symptoms of cystitis. During the taking of a history it is essential to find out exactly what is meant. The term literally means 'inflammation of the bladder' and tells nothing of aetiology. In current medical use it implies frequency of micturition with burning pain in the urethra and perineum. There may also be continuous or intermittent suprapubic pain, low back pain, malaise and urgency of micturition.

Urine is normally sterile. If bacteria enter the bladder and become established, the population doubles every 40 minutes. It follows that the concentration of bacteria can increase rapidly if there is any residual urine in the bladder, or if the times between voids are long (for example, if a patient drinks little).

Bacterial cystitis is nearly always caused by Gram-negative organisms from the intestinal tract. Infection is thought to be by ascent from the perineum. The commonest organism, *E. coli*, forms less than 1 per cent of the faecal bacteria, so there must be special factors that allow it to infect the bladder so frequently. In women suffering recurrent infection the introitus first becomes colonized; the introitus of normal women is colonized much less often. The response to this is a rise in IgA that normally terminates the episode of colonization, and it has been suggested, though not proven, that this response is less efficient in patients becoming infected.

From the introitus, bacteria ascend to the bladder. Deformation of the urethra during intercourse is the most important factor in promoting the ascent; turbulent urine flows in the urethra may be an important factor in the celibate.

On reaching the bladder, the bacteria must reproduce before they are diluted by sterile urine or washed out by voiding. Bacteria reaching the bladder at night – the most usual time for intercourse – will have an advantage. In addition, receptor sites on the cells of the bladder mucosa may allow specific serotypes of *E. coli* to adhere.

Aetiology

Anything that irritates the bladder or urethra, causing local inflammation, can cause the symptoms of cystitis. Patients generally assume that bacterial infection is the cause but, although it is the single most common cause, it only accounts for 35–50 per cent of episodes presenting in general practice. Other causes to be considered include bladder cancer, stones, specific infections (e.g. tuberculosis, schistosomiasis), extravesical lesions (e.g. pelvic inflammatory disease, vaginitis, diverticulitis), urethritis and non-specific problems such as the 'urethral syndrome'.

Bacterial cystitis is most commonly seen in women between the end of puberty and middle age, and attacks often recur. There is a strong association with sexual intercourse, and the condition is often labelled 'honeymoon cystitis'.

History

Obtaining a good history from patients presenting with symptoms of cystitis can be difficult. The chronology must be detailed:

(a) *Patients presenting early with their first attack*: This is the easier group. Patients will be clear when the symptoms began, whether they are continuous day and night, and whether there are systemic symptoms as well. The largest group of patients are teenage girls whose cystitis has been precipitated by their first experiences of sexual intercourse.

Cystitis occurring for no obvious reason in children, any man, or a previously well woman over 50 years, is a worrying event, suggesting a significant underlying lesion.

(b) *Patients presenting with recurrent cystitis*: In addition to the information required from group (a), the age at which the first attack occurred, the periodicity, the results of previous urine cultures, and responses to treatment (especially antibiotics), must be detailed. It is usually possible to separate those with simple bacterial infection from the rest – the former have consistently positive cultures and respond within 24 hours to conventional antibiotics, while the latter have more chronic symptoms. Those with complicated infections may have unusual organisms on culture (e.g. *Proteus*), or respond slowly to antibiotics. Those who have no infection will follow their own natural history uninfluenced by the antibiotics.

Examination

There are usually few physical signs in 'uncomplicated' cystitis. Patients with pyelonephritis will have a tender kidney and signs of systemic infection. Chronic retention of urine is identified by a palpable bladder. The parts of the urinary tract most accessible to examination are the prostate in men and urethra in both sexes: rectal or vaginal examination and examination of the penis is essential. Occult neurological lesions are suggested by abnormalities of the skin over the bottom of the spine, or even palpable bony abnormalities.

Investigation of infected cases

All patients presenting with symptoms of cystitis *must* have their urine

84 Infections of the urinary tract

examined. A mid-stream specimen should be collected in a sterile container and tested with a commercially available dipstick (N-Multistix) to identify the presence of glucose, nitrites, blood and protein. The presence of nitrites is highly suggestive of infection; the presence of protein is not. A stick test for urinary leucocyte esterase has become available recently (Cytur test); a positive result correlates well with the presence of more than 10 leucocytes per millilitre, suggesting significant bacteriuria. Thereafter the material is sent for microscopy and culture. There can be few tests that are so easy for the doctor, painless for the patient and cost-effective in diagnosis. A therapeutic trial of antibiotics is likely to be ineffective in 50–65 per cent of cases.

Significant bacteriuria is defined as the presence of more than 100,000 organisms per millilitre grown in pure culture. Two consecutive mid-stream urine specimens with these features make infection 95 per cent probable. Very dilute urine may occasionally be infected and not fulfil these criteria. Likewise, a pure culture of *Proteus mirabilis*, even with lower concentration, would warrant further investigation, especially if the urinary pH were alkaline (suggesting splitting of urea to release ammonia).

Significant bacteriuria is usually associated with 10 or more leucocytes per high-powered field. In the absence of urinary leucocytes, culture should be repeated before attributing symptoms to bacterial infection.

For patients with proven bacterial cystitis, further investigation depends on the results of urine tests and the clinical problem. Sexually active young women should not be investigated any further for an underlying cause. The following generally should be investigated:

(1) all children, especially those under six years of age;
(2) all men;
(3) all very frequently recurrent cases;
(4) all patients infected with unusual organisms such as *Proteus* or *Pseudomonas*;
(5) all cases of infection that respond poorly to appropriate treatment;
(6) all women presenting with their first infection in middle or old age;

Children

The search is principally for congenital anomalies. As a first screen, patients ideally require a plain abdominal X-ray for bone anomalies and stones; urinary tract ultrasound for deformed kidneys, dilated collecting system and poorly emptying bladder; and micturating cystourethrogram for vesicoureteric reflux.

Men

Young men with urinary tract infection should have an intravenous urogram. If it is normal, further investigation is not indicated, unless there are recurrent infections. The commonest cause of recurrent infections is chronic bacterial prostatitis, which is dealt with later in this chapter.

Frequently recurrent cases, intractable cases, those with unusual organisms, and patients over fifty

In these groups there is a likelihood of an underlying problem. The investigations required depend on the particular clinical suspicion. The first screen should be an intravenous urogram and urine cytology. If these provide no clues, cystoscopy and pelvic examination under general anaesthetic should be done, paying careful attention to the urethra in both sexes. In men, bacterial cystitis may be the first indication of bladder outflow obstruction from prostatic enlargement.

Symptomless bacteriuria

Several studies have shown the prevalence of significant bacteriuria in symptomless schoolgirls (about 1.2 per cent) and in boys (about 0.03 per cent). Bacteriuria in any individual appears and disappears for no apparent reason. Follow-up shows that these children come to no harm and do not develop renal damage. They are said to have occult or symptomless bacteriuria and require no treatment.

In adults, 4 per cent of females and 0.5 per cent of males have symptomless bacteriuria. They are extremely unlikely to develop renal damage, but about one-third will have episodes of symptomatic bacterial cystitis.

It is only in pregnancy, when the kidneys are particularly vulnerable, that symptomless bacteriuria is of importance. The urinary tract, especially the kidneys, is susceptible to bacterial infection in pregnancy. About 20 per cent of patients with bacteriuria will develop pyelonephritis. Regular culture of midstream urine is an essential part of antenatal care.

Management of specific problems of cystitis

It is a very unfortunate fact of life that many women suffer recurrent bacterial cystitis without having any identifiable urinary tract anomaly. It is most commonly associated with sexual intercourse, but it also occurs in the celibate. Other patients may have recurrent infections due to a definable but untreatable cause.

Although none of these patients can be cured, the frequency and severity of attacks can be considerably reduced by careful management. Management may include general measures, adjustment of sexual technique, or the use of antibiotics. The following notes apply to sexually active women, but the general principles apply to other groups.

General measures

General measures are aimed at reducing introital colonization.

Vaginitis, usually fungal in origin, must be identified and treated. Many scented soaps, shampoos, vaginal deodorants and washing powders cause mild inflammation in susceptible individuals. Patients should use pure soap, wash their hair over the sink and avoid other irritants. A moist perineum quickly becomes macerated, allowing bacterial colonization. Clothes that prevent evaporation of sweat – particularly nylon pants and tights – should be avoided.

86 *Infections of the urinary tract*

Patients must have a high fluid intake (3 litres a day is a good target). They must void every 2-3 hours, taking plenty of time; and if the residual volume is known to be large, return to the lavatory for another try 15 minutes later (double micturition). In a few patients, surgery to reduce the residual urine in the collecting system or bladder may be justified.

It is particularly important for women to void 15-20 minutes after intercourse.

Sexual technique

The association of recurrent infection in women with intercourse is established, but the particular aspect responsible is not. It is tempting to blame direct trauma which might 'massage' bacteria up the urethra. Many doctors and patients find the discussion of the minute details of intercourse difficult. Furthermore, there is a danger that inappropriate insistence on the dangers of intercourse will make the woman give up altogether – a course that might cure the cystitis, but raise a number of different problems.

On the assumption that trauma is the main problem, women should be advised to lubricate their vagina with K-Y jelly or baby oil before intercourse. Washing the perineum before intercourse might reduce the introital flora, but this procedure is not of proven value in reducing infections.

Antibiotics

Once it has been established that recurrent cystitis is due to bacterial infection, it is right to prescribe antibiotics for each attack. The patient should have at home a supply of appropriate narrow-spectrum antibiotics (e.g. nitrofurantoin or nalidixic acid) and sterile containers. At the first symptom she should collect a mid-stream specimen and start taking antibiotics. At the next convenient time she should deliver the specimen and collect a new prescription. For uncomplicated infections, a three-day course of antibiotics is sufficient for each episode.

If the infections recur with unacceptable frequency, prophylactic antibiotics are indicated. A quarter of the total daily dose taken at night is usually sufficient.

Prostatitis

Three overlapping diseases of the prostate must be distinguished: acute prostatitis, chronic prostatitis and prostatodynia

Acute prostatitis

Acute prostatitis is an infection of the prostate usually caused by Gram-negative organisms from the large bowel, or *Gonococcus neisseria*. Occasionally it is caused by other organisms such as *Trichomonas* or *Chlamydia*, when urethritis almost invariably occurs as well.

Patients present with an acute febrile illness with severe malaise, rigors, perineal pain and symptoms of cystitis. The prostate is exquisitely tender and swollen, sometimes causing acute retention.

The causative organism can usually be cultured from the first voided urine and sometimes from the blood. Manipulation may cause septicaemia. The prostate should never be massaged in suspected acute prostatitis; instrumentation of the urinary tract should only be done if unavoidable, and then with antibiotic cover.

Treatment is urgent and includes hospitalization, systemic antibiotics (e.g. aminoglycosides) and intravenous fluids. The condition may be complicated by septicaemia or urinary retention.

Chronic prostatitis

This clearly defined condition is frequently and surprisingly confused with prostatodynia and is, therefore, over-diagnosed. It is characterized by recurrent episodes of acute bacterial cystitis which respond to appropriate antibiotics. Between attacks the patient is usually symptomless but may have aching or discomfort in the perineum and mild dysuria. The causative organism can be cultured from prostatic secretions (obtained by massaging the prostate rectally) between attacks.

Although the episodes of cystitis can be treated easily enough, it is very difficult to cure the patient by eradicating the organisms from the prostate. Antibiotics do not penetrate the prostate in sufficient concentration. Short courses of intramuscular amikacin or long courses of cotrimoxazole orally are sometimes effective. Most patients are treated only when they have symptoms, or with low-dose prophylactic antibiotics all the time.

Prostatodynia

This blanket diagnosis is given to men with chronic, non-specific perineal pain. Disease of the prostate, especially carcinoma, diseases elsewhere in the urinary tract and non-urological diseases with referred pain must be carefully excluded before making the diagnosis.

Organisms other than common Gram-negative bacteria (such as *Chlamydia*) have been frequently blamed, but they have rarely been confirmed by appropriate cultures.

There is no specific treatment, and patients present a very difficult management problem.

Many authors have pointed out associations with a range of personality defects and psychiatric illnesses, and psychiatric referral is indicated in severe cases.

Epididymo-orchitis

Bacterial epididymo-orchitis may occur alone, especially in young boys, or as a complication of urinary tract infection. Orchitis alone may occur as part of a generalized viraemia, especially in mumps.

Patients present with an acutely painful and swollen testis, epididymis and scrotum. Proper examination is very difficult, making differentiation from

88 *Infections of the urinary tract*

torsion of the testis virtually impossible. A history of urinary infection, instrumentation or mumps will help.

Only investigations that can be done immediately are justified. Doppler identification of a patent testicular artery or gallium isotope scan may be helpful. If there is doubt about the diagnosis the scrotum should be explored to exclude torsion.

Treatment consists of analgesia, scrotal support and antibiotics. The condition is slow to resolve and treatments should be continued for three weeks.

Renal infections

Pyelonephritis

This condition is due to bacterial inflammation of the epithelial lining of the renal pelvis, which may spread and involve the renal parenchyma. The condition may present as an acute illness; but in some patients who have underlying predisposing factors, chronic pyelonephritis is a separate entity.

Acute pyelonephritis

Bacteria may reach the pelvis of the kidney by several routes. It is thought in most patients there is retrograde passage of bacteria in the urine along the ureter. It is possible that, in the young patient, this can be associated with vesicoureteric reflux. Blood-borne infection is another possibility.

The majority of patients complain of feeling generally unwell or feverish. Associated with pyrexia, rigors may develop. Subjects often complain of loin pain, and on examination the kidney is tender to palpation. Not all patients complain of frequency and dysuria, and indeed the urine is often surprisingly clear. In florid cases the urine may be turbid owing to the high content of inflammatory cells and organisms.

Immediate management may involve analgesia. Certainly antibiotics should be started, and they may have to be given parenterally if the patient is severely ill. Urine should be sent for culture and the antibiotic regimen changed if there is no clinical response and the organisms are resistant to the initial choice of antibiotic.

When the symptoms have subsided, further investigations should include the routine assessment of renal function. An IVU should be performed to ensure that there is no underlying cause (such as a renal calculus) for the infection. Vesicoureteric reflux should be excluded with a micturating cystogram.

Acute pyelonephritis is most common in women. There is, unfortunately, a high recurrence rate in at least 25 per cent of patients.

The common organisms often associated with this condition are *Escherichia coli*, *Streptococcus faecalis*, *Klebsiella*, *Pseudomonas* and *Proteus*. It is possible, by means of ureteric catheterization and sophisticated immunological techniques, to localize the site of infection. It is a surprise that approximately a quarter of the patients in whom these localizing techniques are positive are completely symptom-free.

Chronic pyelonephritis

The most important aetiological factor is the presence of vesicoureteric reflux. The result of infected urine reaching the renal pelvis and passing into the renal parenchyma via incompetent collecting ducts leads to segmental inflammation of the kidney, resulting in damage and scarring. These scars can be seen on the IVU as depressed areas in the cortex and, in extreme cases, there is little renal substance overlying some of the main calyces, which themselves are often clubbed.

The inflammation often starts in childhood and, if it is promptly treated with antibiotics, it is possible to prevent further damage; then, in adult life, if there has not been extensive damage to the kidney, function is often preserved. However, if there has been widespread scarring and loss of functioning renal tissue, there is often a progressive loss of renal function during adult life. This may be compounded by recurrent infection and the development of hypertension.

The clinical picture may be confused with analgesic nephropathy (see pp. 156 and 169), and it is possible that in a certain number of these patients analgesic abuse is responsible for further loss of renal function.

If the condition is unilateral and hypertension is a problem in adult life, then a nephrectomy may be indicated. Before surgery, renal scintigraphy should be performed to ensure that the kidney to be removed is not making the major contribution to the overall function.

Renal abscesses

One-third of all renal abscesses are thought to be caused by circulating bacteria, especially *Staphyloccus aureus*, lodging in the renal parenchyma. They follow a minor and often forgotten injury some days or weeks before presentation. Two-thirds arise from suppuration during acute pyelonephritis.

The condition is rare in Western countries, but the incidence has been rising slowly in recent years, particularly among drug addicts. It is more commonly seen in the malnourished.

The generalized signs of infection from bacteraemia – fever, rigors and sweating – predominate on presentation. The local pain and tenderness from the abscess itself may be overlooked. There are usually no urinary symptoms.

Examination of the urine is unhelpful, except that a few red blood cells may be present. Blood culture is usually positive, and blood count shows a raised white cell count and erythrocyte sedimentation rate (ESR).

Plain abdominal X-rays may show loss of definition of the psoas shadow and scoliosis concave to the affected side. An intravenous urogram shows a non-functioning mass distorting adjacent calyces. The definitive investigation is a renal ultrasound: an abscess is seen as a partly solid, partly cystic lesion that can be difficult to distinguish from a small carcinoma. Under ultrasound guidance the abscess can be needled and pus sent for culture.

A renal arteriogram is often recommended, but this rarely gives more information than ultrasound. The lesion is shown to be displacing blood vessels and calyces but has no tumour circulation. However, in late cases the appearances may be confusing as new vessels grow into the abscess, mimicking a 'tumour circulation'. If there is suspicion that the lesion may be a tumour, it must be needled anyway.

Treatment

After aspiration, treatment with antibiotics for 4 weeks will clear 90 per cent of abscesses with minimal damage to renal function. The progress of treatment should be monitored by serial ultrasound. Surgical drainage is very rarely required, though repeated aspiration is indicated for slow resolution.

Pyonephrosis

Pyonephrosis is an infection of an obstructed renal calyx or pelvis. Infection almost always ascends from the bladder and is, therefore, by Gram-negative organisms.

In contrast to a renal abscess (discussed above), local symptoms and signs predominate. This is an acute, severe illness, and antibiotics rarely penetrate the obstructed system sufficiently to clear the infection.

The cause of the renal obstruction may have made itself known before the onset of infection; for example, the passage of a small stone into the ureter. In other cases, the onset of pyonephrosis may be the first sign that anything is wrong. Twenty per cent of untreated staghorn renal calculi develop pyonephrosis or perinephric abscess.

Onset is rapid with local pain and signs of systemic infection. It may be complicated by Gram-negative septicaemia. In the long term, obstruction complicated by infection will cause progressive renal damage.

The urine contains red and white blood cells. Infection behind a complete obstruction may fail to produce a positive urine culture. Blood culture, on the other hand, is commonly positive. A plain X-ray of the abdomen may show an obstructing stone, and an intravenous urogram shows a non-functioning kidney or, where only one group of calyces is obstructed, a non-functioning area. Renal ultrasound shows a dilated collecting system and distinguishes between obstruction and 'non-function' from other causes.

Treatment

A pyonephrosis is one of the few urological conditions that requires urgent treatment. It is essential to drain the obstruction quickly if any renal function is to be saved. However, once drainage is established and any thick pus washed out, the effluent will be mostly urine, which requires only a very fine gauge tube. The treatment of choice, therefore, is insertion of a small nephrostomy tube percutaneously.

Once the obstructed kidney is draining freely the emergency is over. Antibiotics active against urinary Gram-negative organisms are given – in practice, an aminoglycoside such as gentamicin – until the sensitivities of the bacteria in the aspirated pus are available.

In a few cases, or if facilities for percutaneous needling are not available, it is possible to drain an obstructed kidney by passing a retrograde catheter up the ureter.

The nephrostomy tube *in situ* can be used to define the obstruction radiographically, and to measure the differential creatinine clearance. On this basis a decision on further management can be made. The patient, meanwhile, recovers from the toxic condition in which he or she originally presented. In some cases the track of the nephrostomy tube can be dilated so that the obstruction can be treated by definitive percutaneous surgery (see Chapter 10).

Perinephric abscess

If only a single calyx or group of calyces is affected by pyonephrosis, presentation may be much less dramatic than that described in the previous section. The condition may run an indolent course and avoid receiving early treatment. Sometimes there may be no symptoms at all from a small infected stone obstructing a calyx.

The natural history is one of gradual destruction of surrounding renal parenchyma by a combination of pressure atrophy and suppuration. The abscess extends centrifugally, rarely discharging into the rest of the collecting system, but into the perinephric fat. It thus becomes a perinephric abscess. Eventually it may even present as a fluctuant mass in the flank, usually because it has found its way through the superior lumbar triangle bordered by serratus posterior inferior, the internal oblique and the erector spinae muscles.

Perinephric abscess may also arise by direct spread from an adjacent infection (such as an appendix abscess), or by haematogenous spread from a remote focus.

Treatment

By definition, a perinephric abscess has a chronic presentation. The first step is to drain the abscess. Thereafter, the cause of the obstruction and the residual function of the kidney are defined.

In cases where the renal function has been destroyed, nephrectomy must be done or else the abscess will discharge indefinitely. If there is worthwhile residual function, partial nephrectomy or removing a stone may be possible. Conservative surgery on a kidney that has been bathed in pus for a long time is difficult – and unrewarding as it is seldom possible to preserve renal function.

Genitourinary tuberculosis

Tuberculosis enters at either end of the urinary tract via the blood stream. Thereafter it spreads in the urine or semen.

Virtually all cases have a primary site of infection elsewhere. In Western countries, where bovine infection has been eradicated, the primary site is pulmonary, and the organism is *Mycoplasma tuberculosis*. In underdeveloped countries the primary site may be either pulmonary or gastrointestinal, and so *M. bovis* will be an alternative organism. There is a delay of between 5 and 20 years from the primary to the genitourinary infection: during this time the primary infection may have been treated or healed spontaneously.

Tuberculosis is a common disease in the world and kills between 4 and 5 million people a year. In the United Kingdom the incidence has been falling for many years. About 5 per cent of patients with pulmonary disease develop genitourinary infection, so that each urologist will see only a small number of cases. It is widely known that tuberculosis is common in immigrants, but recently there has been an increase in notifications from the native population. For these reasons the clinician must always be on the lookout so that a serious and curable disease is not missed.

Pathology

In 95 per cent of cases the organisms enter the urinary tract in the kidney. The first lesion is found in the glomeruli, where the organism multiplies to form a granuloma and then a microscopic abscess. Many abscesses heal spontaneously. Others ulcerate into the proximal tubule, releasing the bacillus into the urine. At this stage there is no radiologically detectable lesion, but the organism can be cultured from early-morning urine specimens, which are particularly concentrated.

The micro-abscesses progress centripetally and eventually reach a renal papilla. The papilla becomes necrotic and the abscess opens into the calyx. An intravenous urogram will now show a cavity communicating with the collecting system. Renal tuberculosis should always be regarded as multifocal and bilateral.

In the early stages renal destruction is a direct effect of the bacteria. By the time the disease has broken through to the collecting system, the process consists of a mixture of destruction and healing by fibrosis. The fibrosis causes strictures, usually of the calyceal necks, which obstruct parenchymal drainage and accelerate the destruction. In this phase part or all of the kidney may be silently destroyed, often with secondary calcification. Remission may occur at any time, so that apparently fit people are occasionally seen who have a non-functioning and calcified kidney on one side due to earlier tuberculous infection – a so-called 'autonephrectomy'. Calcification does not necessarily imply healing: calcified lesions are indeed thought to have a worse prognosis.

Further foci of infection can occur in the ureter, especially at the sites of relative narrowing: the pelvic brim and the ureterovesical junction. The resulting strictures cause further pressure atrophy of the kidney.

In the bladder the first lesions are always seen around the ureteric orifices, spreading to produce generalized involvement. The end result is a shrunken, fibrosed bladder with small capacity and a stiff (hypocompliant) wall.

The route of infection of the lower genitourinary tract is unknown. The fact that about 30 per cent of cases of tuberculous prostatitis occur without other urinary tract infection suggests that blood-borne spread is possible. Infection of the epididymis does not occur in isolation, but may be a site of florid presentation. There is usually generalized infection of the male genital tract: the obstructing lesions cause infertility in nearly all cases.

The slowly destructive lesions of tuberculosis produce necrotic debris and pools of static urine. It is not surprising, therefore, that secondary infections with common Gram-negative pathogens, such as *E. coli*, are common. In cultures only the *E. coli* will grow. The correct diagnosis will only be made if frequently recurrent cases of UTI are adequately investigated.

Presentations

The discovery of a partly calcified renal lesion on an abdominal X-ray or pyuria with negative culture for conventional urinary pathogens (sterile pyuria) are the commonest chance presentations. Some cases are found during routine follow-up of known pulmonary cases.

Frequently recurrent episodes of urinary tract infection and haematuria should provoke further investigation. Persistent pyuria after successful clearance of the presenting pathogen and discontinuation of antibiotics raises the suspicion of underlying disease. An intravenous urogram and urine cultures for tuberculosis are indicated.

So far as local symptoms are concerned, the hallmark of tuberculosis is painless destruction. Painless but severe frequency will follow fibrosis and shrinkage of the bladder. Slow, painless enlargement of the epididymis is the most important scrotal sign: ultimately a sinus may develop.

Investigations

In most cases a urine sample contains an excess of white cells. Rarely, there may only be a few red cells or some proteinuria. The tubercle bacillus is acid and alcohol fast on staining (Ziel–Nielson staining technique). Unfortunately the number of organisms present in any lesion is very small and so they are difficult to find in the urine. At least three early-morning specimens of urine must be examined. If they are negative and clinical suspicion is strong, a further three or even six specimens will have to be examined before tuberculosis can be excluded. The smegma bacillus is also acid and alcohol fast. Mycobacterium grows very slowly in culture. Even in heavily infected urine, colonies take three weeks to develop. With a small initial inoculum culture may take 6–8 weeks.

There are no specific blood tests for tuberculosis. The ESR is usually raised and its subsequent measurement is a useful monitor of successful treatment.

Calcified lesions may be seen on a plain abdominal X-ray. On IVU there is little to see in early cases. Later, small cavities communicating with the collecting system are seen, most commonly in the upper pole. Progressive disease is seen as ever-larger cavities. 'Burnt out' disease or autonephrectomy is indicated by a small calcified non-functioning kidney. If the ureter is affected, fibrosis causes stricture with proximal dilatation. The bladder appears normal, except in very late cases when it is shrunken.

Cystoscopy is not necessary in early cases confirmed by culture. If there is diagnostic doubt, cystoscopy for mucosal biopsy may be helpful.

Treatment

All cases are treated with triple therapy at first. Regimens are being refined all the time. Isoniazid, rifampicin, ethambutol and pyrazinamide are the most

94 Infections of the urinary tract

effective drugs; 3-6 months is the commonest treatment period, though some centres are still giving as much as 12-18 months of treatment. Patients on ethambutol require careful supervision by an ophthalmologist as over-dosage may be complicated by blindness.

Lesions healing during treatment become fibrosed, and silent strictures occur to cause renal obstruction. Kidneys must be monitored, preferably by ultrasound, at least weekly during the first month of treatment.

Surgical treatment is needed less and less often. Ureteric strictures are excised. Completely closed cavities in the renal parenchyma occasionally require excision, but only if medical treatment fails to heal them.

In very late cases a shrunken bladder, causing severe frequency, may be removed and replaced by a length of caecum. When the bladder is removed, the trigone and a rim of bladder anteriorly are preserved and the caecum is isolated from the gastrointestinal tract and sutured on (caecocystoplasty). Most patients void normally thereafter, but some need to catheterize themselves.

10
Obstruction

Urinary tract obstruction is a common clinical problem and represents an area of nephrology where recent advances in diagnosis and treatment have reduced morbidity. The obstruction can be complete and sudden and the patient will pass no urine (anuria), or a partial obstruction may develop over months and is often associated with an increased urine production (polyuria) despite a fall in glomerular filtration rate.

An understanding of the pathophysiology allows a clearer interpretation of the patient's signs and symptoms and helps with the assessment of subsequent investigations. If the ureter of an experimental animal is ligated the pressure in the renal pelvis rises immediately and then, within hours, falls to normal. This is due to a reduction in the rate of glomerular filtration following the rise in back pressure. There is evidence to suggest that the filtrate is reabsorbed from the renal pelvis and a reduction in muscle tone tends to bring the pressure back to normal. This fall in muscle tone is more marked when the urine is infected. Therefore in the early stages of obstruction the pelvis and calyces are distended and the hydrostatic pressure is high, a situation which can be easily recognized with both invasive and non-invasive techniques; but long-standing obstruction may be more difficult to recognize when the pressure has fallen towards normal and the collecting systems have collapsed. Systemic hypertension may often be a complicating factor but may disappear when the obstruction is relieved.

The amount of permanent damage depends on the degree and duration of the obstruction, with infection being a poor prognostic feature. There is no guide to potential function, and so in order to provide the best chance of recovery, early diagnosis and treatment are essential.

Signs and symptoms

Pain is often a predominant feature, the details of which are found when the various sites of obstruction are discussed. It is important to realize, however, that obstruction, especially if partial, may be silent, with the patient being symptom-free. Clinical examination may reveal a tender, enlarged kidney, a palpable bladder or an enlarged prostate, and it is the following investigations that define the site and cause of obstruction.

Urine analysis

Microscopic haematuria may be associated with stones or malignancy, and the latter may be confirmed by cytology. Proteinuria up to 3-4 g per 24 hours is predominantly due to back-pressure damage on the glomeruli. The presence of infection is an important clinical feature.

Radiology

A plain film with tomography will allow the size of the kidney to be assessed. A large kidney would be compatible with obstruction (a large kidney has to be

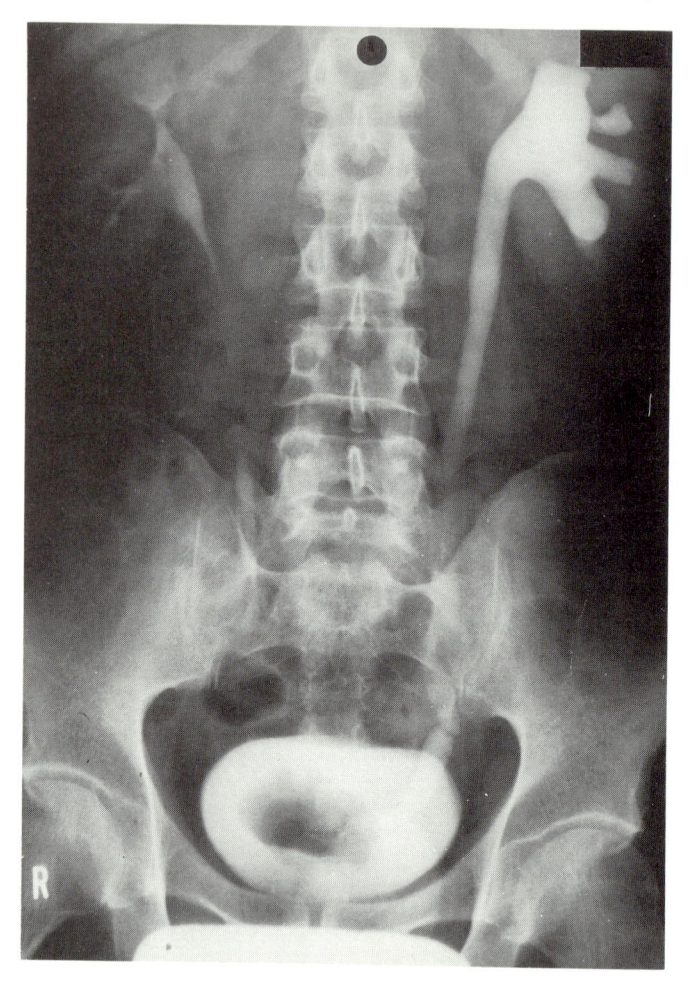

Fig. 10.1 Intravenous urogram in a patient with obstruction of the left kidney and ureter by a stone at the lower end of the ureter. Note the distended left ureter and the 'clubbing' of the calyces compared with the concave shape of the calyces in the (right) unobstructed kidney.

distinguished from enlargement due to infiltration with amyloid or myeloma), and a radio-opaque calculus may be visible. An IVU using double doses of isotonic contrast media may demonstrate the site of obstruction (Fig. 10.1), but exposures as late as 24–36 hours may be required before any pyelogram or ureteric anatomy is defined. Antegrade or retrograde examination of the renal pelvis may not only define the site of obstruction, but will also allow the system to be drained – an important part of early management.

Ultrasound

This non-invasive investigation may well define kidney size and detect the site of obstruction.

Isotopic studies

Probe renography or the use of renal scintigraphy may produce the classical pictures of obstruction (Figs. 10.2 and 10.3). If, however, the obstruction has been prolonged and filtration has ceased, it is impossible to make the diagnosis by the use of this technique.

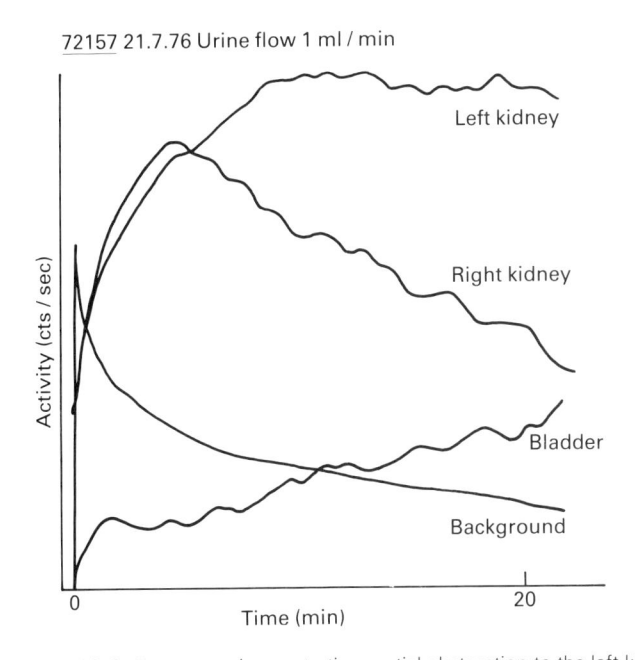

Fig. 10.2 Renogram demonstrating partial obstruction to the left kidney. During the 20 minutes of observation the isotope is cleared rapidly from the right kidney but hardly at all from the left. Isotope accumulates only slowly in the bladder. This renogram was performed in the patient whose IVU is shown in Fig. 10.1.

98 *Obstruction*

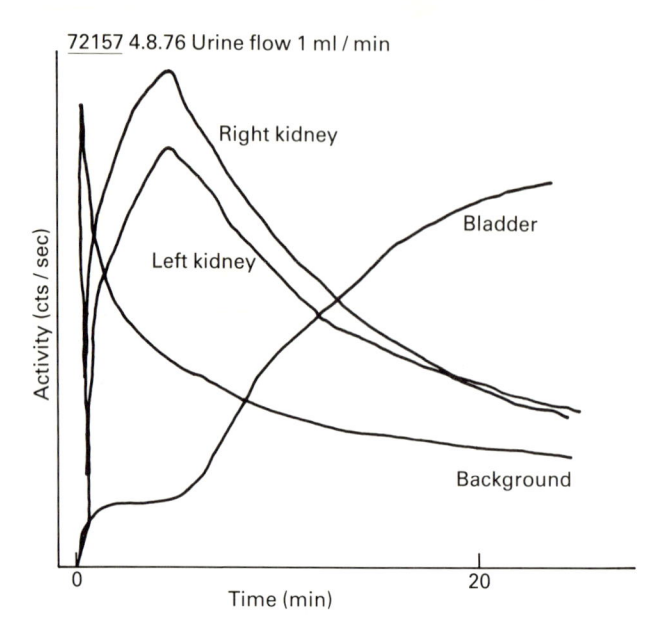

Fig. 10.3 One month after Figs. 10.1 and 10.2 were obtained, the patient's stone has passed spontaneously and the left upper urinary tract is no longer obstructed. Note that contrast leaves the left kidney as rapidly as it does the right, and that accumulation of contrast in the bladder is now rapid.

Kidney obstruction

Stones

Stones less than 3 mm in diameter commonly pass from the kidney causing severe, colicky pain. They may be held up at the pelviuretic junction, causing an obstruction. Stones between 3 and 5 mm may pass spontaneously.

Stones over 5 mm may obstruct a calyceal neck. In this site they are usually painless. They cause back pressure on the nephrons draining into that calyx. The stagnant pool of urine thus formed provides ideal conditions for further growth of the stone.

If the stone escapes from the calyx it may impact permanently or temporarily at the pelviureteric junction. This is painful and causes back pressure on the whole kidney.

In some patients, particularly those infected with urea-splitting organisms such as *Proteus mirabilis*, stones may grow silently to fill the renal collecting system completely. The branched form gives them the name 'staghorn' calculi. They destroy the kidney through a combination of pressure and infection.

Treatment

Single small stones may cause no symptoms or renal damage. They may be safely left alone. Patients should have a plain X-ray and urine culture each year: stone growth or urine infection are indications for removal.

Small stones causing pain should be removed. It can be very difficult to find a small stone at open operation, even when peroperative X-ray is available. The new technique of stone removal by nephroscope through a percutaneous tract is simpler for patient and surgeon.

Large stones and staghorns are removed at open operation. Every effort must be made to preserve the kidney unless its function is below 10 per cent of the total.

Non-operative treatment by extracorporeal shock-wave lithotripsy is now available in some centres and its use will increase. The stone is fragmented by a focussed shock wave and the particles are passed down the ureter.

Necrotic papillae

In papillary necrosis (Hladky and Rink, p. 124), papillae may detach. Those that have become calcified may obstruct the renal pelvis and require removal.

Pelviureteric junction obstruction

Although structural abnormalities can be found with electron microscopy, PUJ obstruction is best regarded as a disorder of function. The junction is unable to transmit boluses of urine from the pelvis into the ureter. During periods of high urine production more is produced than can be transported, leading to an intra-renal pressure rise. Surprisingly this is often painless, though some patients complain of an ache and fewer still of the 'classical' symptom of pain after drinking large quantities of beer. During periods of low urine production the transmission mechanism at the PUJ may be able to cope, so that obstruction is intermittent.

It is probably a congenital abnormality and can be bilateral. Presentation is usually in childhood or adolescence, though it is possible at any age.

Treatment

Possible cases must be carefully investigated. Dilatation of the renal pelvis on conventional intravenous urography is not synonymous with obstruction. Pressure measurements from within the renal pelvis may be required to confirm significant obstruction. In established obstruction, reconstruction of the junction to make a 'funnel' shape is curative (Fig. 10.4).

Strictures

Strictures of the calyceal necks are usually tuberculous. True stricture of the PUJ (as opposed to functional obstruction) is usually secondary to stones or surgery.

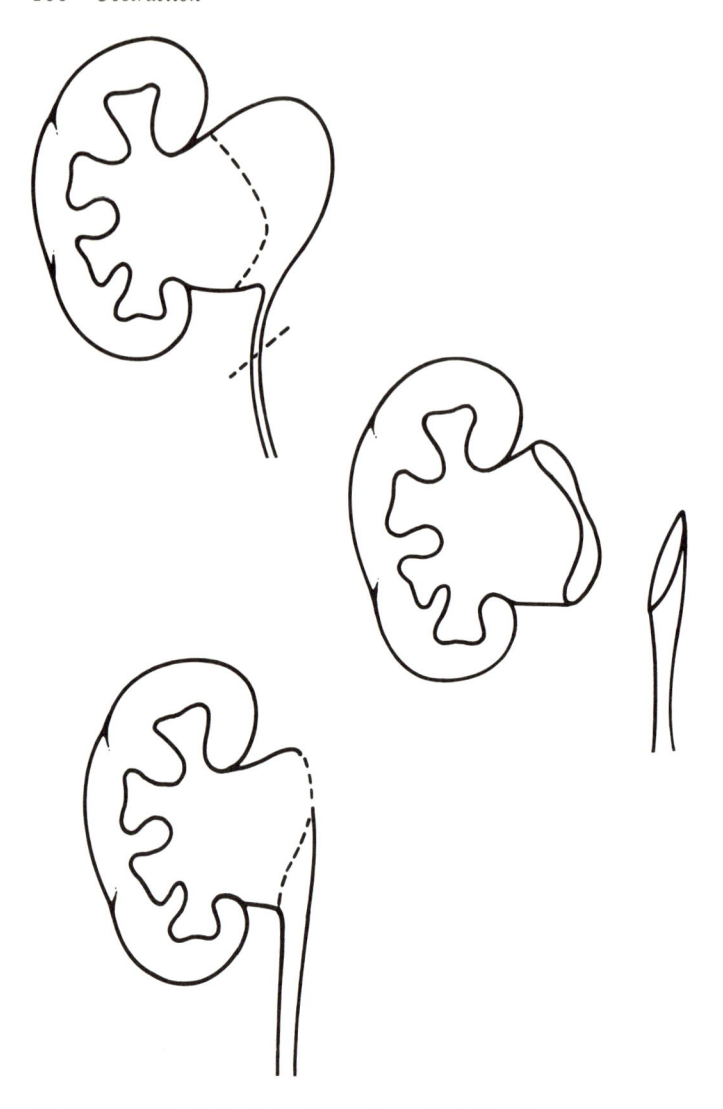

Fig. 10.4 Pelviureteric obstruction and a method of repair.

Tumours

Adenocarcinomas of the kidney impair function by direct destruction of renal parenchyma. Tumours of the epithelial lining of kidney (transitional cell carcinoma) can obstruct calyces or the PUJ, especially if they invade the submucosa. (See Chapter 17.)

Extramural lesions

Isolated obstruction of the renal pelvis by extramural lesions is rare. Any inflammatory or neoplastic lesion in the retroperitoneum could obstruct the kidney, but this is a rare clinical problem.

An artery to the lower pole of the kidney has been blamed for PUJ obstruction. It is not thought now to be a primary cause. However, if a dilated renal pelvis herniates between the main and lower pole arteries, a pre-existing obstruction may be worsened.

Ureteric obstruction

Stones

Stones small enough to pass through the pelviureteric junction will usually pass down the ureter, causing severe pain. The pain is felt in the back on the appropriate side and radiates through the loin and iliac fossa to the tip of the urethra. Bilateral or mid-line back pain is not caused by renal or ureteric disease.

The narrowest parts of the ureter occur at the pelvic brim and where it passes obliquely through the wall of the bladder. Stones may be held up at these points transiently or permanently.

Treatment

This should be conservative. Renal and ureteric colic are very painful and large doses of analgesia are required (e.g. pethidine 100 mg intramuscularly). All patients should have urine microscopy and culture and a plain abdominal X-ray on presentation. If a stone is seen, its progress down the ureter can be followed with serial plain films. If no stone is seen or if the diagnosis is in doubt, an intravenous urogram should be done as an emergency, but otherwise it can be left until the next working day.

The clinician and patient must be prepared to wait (often for several days) as at least 75 per cent of ureteric stones less than 3 mm in diameter will pass spontaneously. High fluid intake will help, but smooth-muscle relaxants do not and may even paralyse the ureter sufficiently to slow down the stone's progress.

Surgical removal is indicated as an emergency if infection occurs in the obstructed kidney and ureter. A small catheter is passed percutaneously into the renal pelvis under X-ray control. This will allow pus and urine to drain. Antibiotics are given. When the patient's general condition has improved, the stone is removed.

If the stone fails to pass after several months or is causing intractable pain, it should be removed. Traditionally, those above the ischial spine are removed by open operation and those below are removed endoscopically by passing a Dormia basket up the ureter. Recent developments now allow almost all ureteric stones to be removed endoscopically: those in the uppermost quarter can be approached percutaneously across the renal pelvis, and those below can be grasped under direct vision using an operating rigid ureteroscope.

Ureteric tumours

Ureteric tumours are rare and arise from the transitional cell epithelium. Associated bladder or renal transitional cell carcinoma should always be expected. The ureter is usually obstructed gradually and without pain. The commonest presentation is with haematuria.

Although only 2 per cent are bilateral, the condition may be multifocal: advanced and invasive cases require radical surgery (such as nephroureterectomy), while early cases require conservative resection. A constant watch must be kept for tumours arising elsewhere in the urinary tract.

Retroperitoneal fibrosis

This is a rare and interesting condition in which the peritoneum of the posterior abdominal wall becomes thickened and fibrotic. The migraine medication methysergide, now obsolete, used to be a common cause. The majority of cases are idiopathic. Malignant retroperitoneal fibrosis occurs *de novo* or with intraabdominal carcinoma or lymphoma.

The disease begins as a plaque of fibrosis which spreads on each side from the level of the renal hilum to the bladder. The ureters are obstructed but not invaded.

Patients present either with back pain or with the complications of bilateral obstruction, such as renal failure or hypertension. The ESR is invariably raised. Intravenous urography shows bilateral obstruction, usually with dilated ureters which are seen to have no peristalsis on screening. It is characteristic that retrograde catheters can be passed freely up to the renal pelves.

Urgent treatment may be required for renal failure, usually by catheter drainage of the renal pelves. Idiopathic retroperitoneal fibrosis will respond to steroids, and progress can be monitored by renal function improving and return of the ESR to normal. However, surgical biopsy is needed to confirm the diagnosis: once the abdomen has been opened, surgical relief of the problem is sensible and avoids the long-term complications of steroids. The ureters are dissected free of the fibrosis and wrapped in greater omentum to prevent recurrence.

Bladder obstruction

Tumours

The bladder is such a large hollow organ that intraluminal and extramural lesions have little chance of obstructing the kidneys. The ureters enter the bladder only 3–4 cm apart, so that tumours of the bladder base are likely to obstruct both. Carcinoma of the bladder or carcinoma of the prostate invading the bladder base is the commonest culprit.

Patients presenting in renal failure from this cause are very difficult management problems. They have the problems both of renal failure and of advanced malignancy. Those who have had no previous treatment for their carcinoma should have bilateral percutaneous nephrostomies made. The extent and nature of the bladder tumour can be investigated at leisure before starting treatment. If, on the other hand, the patient has already exhausted the reasonable therapeutic options for the malignancy, it may be best to offer no treatment: death from renal failure may be preferable to death from recurrent pelvic malignancy.

In the heat of an emergency presentation this can be a very difficult decision to take. Unfortunately, once nephrostomies are made it is very difficult to remove them, because of the risks of persistent urinary fistula and emotional upset.

Bladder neck obstruction

Obstruction at bladder neck level will lead to hypertrophy of the detrusor muscle and therefore to raised intravesical pressure. The pressure will be transmitted back to the kidneys if the junction between ureters and bladder is incompetent. Furthermore, the bands of hypertrophied detrusor muscle may obstruct the ureters in their intramural course.

Bladder neck obstruction of this severity occurs almost exclusively in children. It is functional rather than anatomical: the bladder neck muscle fails to relax during voiding. In early cases there may be nothing to see, but later the bladder neck muscle becomes hypertrophied. However, the diagnosis can only be confirmed by synchronous cystogram and bladder pressure measurements (videocystometrogram).

Bladder neck obstruction may present in adult life but is very rarely of sufficient severity to obstruct the kidneys.

Treatment

The bladder neck is incised transurethrally. The decision to perform this operation must only be taken after full investigation, as it will lead to retrograde ejaculation and sterility in 10 per cent of cases.

Prostate enlargement

Men with enlargement of the prostate commonly present with disordered bladder emptying (see Chapter 11). A small number, however, develop chronic, painless retention of urine. This occurs when the power of the detrusor muscle fails to compensate for the decreasing diameter of the outlet. The bladder slowly distends. The intravesical pressure is low except when the bladder is almost full, at which time the patient can void and partly empty the bladder. He may remain symptomless until bladder sensation is lost and he voids unknowingly, the condition of overflow incontinence.

If the ureterovesical junction is incompetent the ureters, and ultimately the kidney, will dilate. Even though the pressure is low it is sufficient to cause gradual obstruction. Patients present in renal failure with anaemia.

Examination at any time reveals an enlarged bladder which is painless – the essential difference between acute and chronic retention. When chronic renal failure has begun, its physical signs will be apparent (see Chapter 4). Rectal examination confirms an enlarged prostate, but the degree of enlargement is unrelated to the degree of obstruction.

Treatment

Chronic retention, with or without renal failure, requires urgent but not emergency treatment. If the blood urea concentration is grossly raised, a urethral catheter is passed. Unless the kidneys have been damaged beyond all redemption the function will rapidly improve. When the patient is fit enough, the prostate is resectioned transurethrally.

If the blood urea is normal, a catheter should not be passed as this introduces an unnecessary risk of infection. Prostatectomy should be performed at the next convenient opportunity.

The most difficult part of treatment is to restore detrusor muscle tone. It normally returns after catheterization for between 1 and 6 weeks, but a few patients may never regain normal bladder function. Oral distigmine bromide may stimulate detrusor contraction.

Obstructive lesions in children

The genitourinary tract is the commonest site of congenital deformities. Obstructive lesions occur at the pelviureteric junction, the lower end of the ureter, the bladder neck and, in boys, the urethra.

Severe lesions occurring *in utero* prevent full development of the kidneys, so that the infant is born with irreversible renal failure. Milder lesions present in the neonatal period or early years of childhood. Early diagnosis and treatment are critical because the growing kidney is quickly and irreversibly damaged by obstruction.

The problem is compounded by infection which is easily introduced by ill-advised instrumentation. This subject is covered in Chapter 9.

Medical management

Irrespective of the cause and site of the obstruction, the medical management must be concerned with a number of common problems.

If the patient is completely anuric and there has been elevation of blood urea and plasma potassium concentrations, then supportive dialysis may be required to make the patient fit to withstand anaesthesia and surgery. This supportive therapy may be needed in the postoperative period until function returns. In some cases the relief of obstruction is associated with an obligatory loss of sodium and water, and this postoperative diuresis requires careful fluid and sodium replacement. If this is not adequate and started early, hypovolaemia and hypotension with possible further associated renal damage may occur.

It is clearly important to recognize obstruction early as it is only by early diagnosis and surgical relief that renal function may be preserved.

Renal calculi are a common cause of obstruction. Once surgical relief is achieved the aetiology must be considered and appropriate medical treatment commenced. The mixed calcium, magnesium, ammonium phosphate stones associated with infection and obstruction have been considered, and the relief of obstruction and the eradication of infection are central to these patients' management. The metabolic problems associated with renal tubular acidosis, uric acid and cystine metabolism are all described in Chapter 14. This covers the majority of stones that are likely to be met in clinical practice, with the possible exception of the radio-opaque stones associated with pure calcium oxalate. These patients excrete excess oxalate in their urine owing to excessive production. This is due to a specific enzyme defect which may be partially corrected by the oral administration of pyridoxine. A second group of patients with hyperoxaluria are those who have undergone resection of small bowel, and this is thought to be due to excessive absorption of oxalate by the colon. The abnormalities of calcium metabolism which may produce stone disease are covered in *Clinical Endocrinology* by P. Daggett.

11
Disorders of bladder function

Normal bladder function

The bladder has two functions: to store urine and, at an appropriate time, to evacuate it. As the bladder fills with urine the detrusor muscle of the bladder wall relaxes, allowing distension without a rise in pressure. At the end of filling the intrinsic intravesical pressure should be less than 15 cm of water. The first desire to void is usually felt at about two-thirds of capacity but is easily suppressed.

Voiding is initiated by a reflex arc in the spinal cord but with promoting and inhibiting influences from the brain. The detrusor muscle contracts and the two urethral sphincters relax to empty the bladder. The detrusor contraction is maintained to the end of voiding, leaving no residual urine. The intravesical pressure during voiding (voiding pressure: VP) and the flow rate must be considered together, but normally the VP is less than 45 cm of water with a peak flow rate of at least 18 ml/second. The normal bladder capacity is age-dependent and in adults is 300–500 ml.

This very simple description disguises one of the most complicated neurophysiological systems of the body. The anatomical pathways, neural transmitters and control of bladder and urethral function are still disputed.

The filling phase

Experimental evidence and surgical experience with partial cystectomy suggest that filling sensation is felt by stretch receptors in the trigone. Afferent impulses travel in the pelvic sympathetic nerves to the lateral columns on both sides of the spinal cord. There are stretch receptors throughout the bladder. Other receptors for pain, touch and temperature are present, but they are unimportant in the normal bladder. The urgent, almost painful, desire to void experienced with a very full bladder arises from stretch receptors in the proximal urethra which are stimulated when the bladder neck opens.

The filling phase is continuous as urine is produced all the time. Obviously the bladder stores urine but not as a static condition, the wall progressively relaxing to accommodate the increasing volume. The capacity of the bladder is ultimately controlled by the elastic properties of the bladder wall and by the

Normal bladder function 107

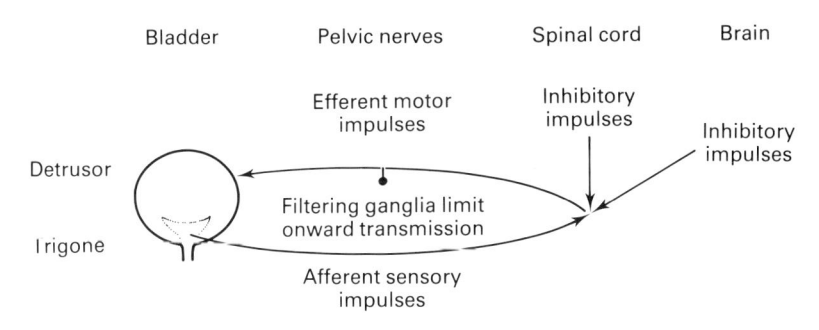

```
           Bladder      Pelvic nerves      Spinal cord       Brain

                        Efferent motor     Inhibitory
                        impulses           impulses        Inhibitory
Detrusor                                                   impulses
                        Filtering ganglia limit
                        onward transmission
Trigone
                        Afferent sensory
                        impulses
```

Fig. 11.1 Neural impulses in bladder filling.

ability to suppress efferent impulses to the detrusor muscle generated by the afferent input from bladder filling. Suppression is achieved by inhibitory impulses produced within the spinal cord in response to filling, by the failure of some 'filtering' ganglia to transmit the efferent impulses, and by inhibitory impulses from the brain (Fig. 11.1). The inhibitory activity is suppressed at the end of filling so that voiding may be initiated.

The urethra responds to filling of the bladder by increased sphincter activity, which increases the urethral pressure. The pelvic floor muscles respond to rises in intravesical and intra-abdominal pressure by contracting which lengthens the urethra, thus further increasing the urethral pressure. So long as this mechanism is working, sudden rises in intra-abdominal pressure – from coughing, sneezing, lifting and running – do not cause incontinence.

The initiation of voiding

The first act of voiding is a fall in the urethral pressure. This will happen automatically when the bladder is completely filled, but the mechanism of its initiation in normal life is unknown. There is certainly a reflex element in response to bladder filling and a central element from the brain.

The centres for the voluntary control of micturition are in the superior frontal gyrus, anterior cingulate gyrus and the genu of the corpus callosum which lie in the medial part of the frontal lobe. However, there are other cortical centres involved and it is not yet clear which are initiating and which inhibitory. The centre responsible for the striated pelvic floor muscle is in the paracentral lobule of the pre- and post-central gyrus: it is an initiating centre, and lesions in this area cause inability of the pelvic floor to relax and prevent the urethra opening.

The fall in urethral pressure is accompanied by the urgent sensation that voiding is about to occur and is followed within a few seconds by detrusor contraction. The detrusor is innervated by the parasympathetic system, nerves arising in S3 and 4 and travelling in the pelvic plexus to ganglia on and within the bladder wall. Although the nerves are parasympathetic, the detrusor muscle does not behave as it should with purely, cholinergic innervation. Experimental and electron-microscopic studies suggest that there is another neuromuscular transmitter which is non-cholinergic and non-adrenergic. There are several

108 *Disorders of bladder function*

candidates for this role, and it is most likely to be a neuropeptide such as VIP (vasoactive intestinal peptide) or substance P.

Sympathetic nerves to the bladder and urethra arise from T10 to L2 and also join the pelvic plexus. Adrenergic nerve endings are seen in greatest number in the bladder neck area in males and are relatively scanty in females. The sympathetic system probably has no direct role in the voiding cycle; the wide interconnections with the parasympathetic ganglia suggest that its function may be to modify parasympathetic activity. In males it may act to close the bladder neck during ejaculation.

Voiding

The beginning of detrusor contraction coincides with the opening of the bladder neck. The mechanism of bladder neck opening is another unknown factor in the complex action. It may be an entirely passive movement resulting from raised intravesical pressure, though this seems unlikely as abdominal wall contraction alone does not open it; it may be pulled open by contraction of radially lying detrusor fibres; or it may occur by relaxation of separately innervated circumferential bladder neck fibres.

The urethra shortens with relaxation of the periurethral muscles. The circular fibres of the external sphincter also relax to widen the urethral lumen.

Because the detrusor muscle contracts before the full length of the urethra is open, the bladder pressure is high at the onset of micturition. Furthermore, the force exerted by the muscle fibres is proportional to their length at the beginning of contraction (up to a certain maximum). Therefore, at the beginning of micturition the flow rate is at its greatest and, within reason, the fuller the bladder, the greater the flow.

In some normal people, mainly women, contraction of the abdominal wall contributes to voiding. It is a relatively inefficient method of voiding because it fails to open the bladder neck completely and, indeed, some of the pressure generated is applied to the upper urethra, thus keeping it closed. If the detrusor fails, the abdominal wall is a very unsatisfactory substitute.

The resistance to flow offered by the urethra is a critical factor in urology and the subject of much research. The diameter is variable throughout its length, especially in the male: however, in most men a sound of at least 7-8 mm diameter (22 French gauge) will pass freely into the bladder. In full flow the diameter is only about 3-4 mm. A considerable 'anatomical' narrowing is therefore required before the flow rate is reduced, but the flow characteristics may be changed by even quite minor strictures.

Obstructions to outflow

Because of the considerable 'reserve' in outflow diameter, obstruction tends to occur insidiously. Except in a few rare congenital lesions, it almost never occurs in females and all of the following comments refer to men. The only symptom that outflow obstruction causes directly is diminished stream: the other symptoms are due to secondary effects on the rest of the system, especially the detrusor muscle.

Benign prostatic hypertrophy (BPH)

Growth of the prostate is best regarded as part of the normal ageing process. Increase in size may obstruct the lumen of the urethra and thus diminish flow. The degree of obstruction, however, is not related to the size achieved: huge prostates of 100 g or more may cause no symptoms, while small, fibrous glands of 20 g may produce complete obstruction.

As a general rule, the more proximal the obstruction to bladder outflow, the more severe are the secondary effects. The detrusor, in most cases, responds to a smaller outflow by contracting harder, the muscle fibres becoming hypertrophied. During this compensated phase there are usually no symptoms. About 50 or 60 per cent of men will then develop *unstable detrusor contractions*: the detrusor contracts spontaneously before the bladder is full and normal reflex and conscious inhibitory mechanisms fail to suppress it. These waves of contraction are felt as an urgent desire to void, especially if they are powerful enough to open the bladder neck. They are seen on a cystometrogram as spikes of high detrusor pressure which interrupt the normal pattern of filling, and are usually associated with an end filling pressure of above 15 cm of water. In severe cases the detrusor pressure exceeds the urethral pressure and the patient is incontinent – so-called 'urge incontinence'.

Detrusor instability reduces the functional capacity of the bladder. The triad of symptoms produced – urgency, frequency and nocturia – are often called 'prostatism'. This unsatisfactory term should be abandoned: detrusor instability is a common response to a variety of disorders, not all of which are obstructive. Many urological disasters have been caused by prostatectomy performed for these symptoms alone.

The hypertrophy of the detrusor muscle from any cause is seen as randomly arranged bands in the bladder wall – *trabeculation*. With time the muscle is partly replaced by interstitial collagen which diminishes the compliance of the bladder wall and its power to contract. The finding of gross trabeculation on cystoscopy is not an indication of a powerful muscular organ but of an effete one that is long past its prime. In a few cases the mucosa is herniated out between the muscle bundles first as saccules and then as diverticula. Large bladder diverticula, having no muscle wall, empty poorly and are thus common sites for infection and stone formation. They increase any post-voiding residual and further decrease the detrusor efficiency.

A characteristic symptom of prostatic enlargement is *hesitancy*: an embarrassing delay between opening the trousers and the start of voiding. The cause of this symptom is not certain, but is probably failure of the urethra to open, rather than of the detrusor to contract.

Instability is not, of course, the only pathway that the bladder may take in response to prostatic enlargement. *Acute retention* may occur at any stage of the process, but is commonest early on, often before other symptoms have become apparent. It is, by definition, painful, though the intravesical pressure is not particularly high – usually between 30 and 40 cm of water. The immediate cause is usually stretching of the detrusor fibres beyond the point that contraction is possible. Precipitating factors include excess alcohol intake which dulls the senses and increases urine production, delayed voiding due to social

110 *Disorders of bladder function*

circumstances, drug ingestion, severe illness or sexual activity. Occasionally, sudden increase in prostatic size such as occurs with acute prostatitis may precipitate retention.

Acute retention may be relieved by passage of a small catheter: if the catheter is removed after the bladder is emptied, at least 50 per cent of patients are able to void normally, but will have further episodes of retention. A single episode in a patient with BPH is usually taken as an indication for prostatectomy.

In units with a well-trained staff the passage of a small suprapubic catheter (such as a Bonano) is preferable to a urethral one. It saves the risk of urethral stricture; allows trial of voiding merely by clamping the catheter; and allows drainage during and after prostatectomy. A suprapubic catheter should not be passed unless the bladder is palpable suprapubically; another contraindication is a previous lower abdominal operation.

In a third group of patients, the bladder enters a phase of *decompensation*. The failure of the bladder to reach its optimal volume before voiding starts leads to a slower peak flow rate and a prolonged void, even though the voided volume is small. The detrusor muscle later fails to maintain its contraction, generating a low pressure and leaving a residual volume in the bladder (which may or may not give rise to a sensation of incomplete emptying). In extreme cases chronic painless retention develops – the patient voids, or is incontinent of, small volumes only at the extreme of bladder filling.

A residual urine predisposes to bacterial infection, so that acute cystitis may be a presenting symptom. Cystitis may also cause acute retention superimposed on pre-existing chronic retention.

The ureters and kidneys are protected from the transient rises in intravesical pressure that occur in bladder outflow obstruction by the competence of the ureterovesical junction. In chronic retention the junction may become incompetent, the pressure transmitted upwards and renal function impaired. Patients may present with painless retention, advanced renal failure and anaemia.

Investigations

In the majority of patients a diagnosis of benign prostatic hypertrophy is easy enough from the history of outflow symptoms, secondary effects on the bladder and digital examination of the prostate. If the diagnosis is in doubt, especially in a patient under 55 years, videocystometry is indicated (see Chapter 2). Prostatectomy should not be performed for frequency alone.

The role of other investigations is less clear. The high incidence of bacteriuria and the cheapness of the investigation makes microscopy and culture of midstream urine obligatory. No patient should undergo major surgery without having a haemoglobin test and an estimation of renal function. The IVU will not pick up any more abnormalities in BPH patients than in a group of age-matched but symptomless men: it is, therefore, difficult to justify its routine use on scientific grounds. Nonetheless, many urologists feel that the IVU has a well-established role in the investigation of urological patients and are unwilling to give it up.

Prostatectomy

The treatment of outflow obstruction from BPH is removal of the enlarged part of the prostate. The operation may be done under general or regional anaesthesia. The urethra and bladder are inspected with a cystoscope first and any coincidental lesions dealt with. The size of the prostate is then assessed bimanually.

The risk of complications and suffering of the patient are so much reduced by transurethral resection (TUR) as opposed to open operation that this must be the method of choice unless there are very compelling reasons to the contrary. Excessive size of the gland is the only important contraindication to TUR, and even this is not an absolute criterion, depending on the skill of the surgeon and the condition of the patient. A transuretheral resection lasting more than about 75–90 minutes has a high risk of fluid overload (see below). In this time a urologist can resect about 100 g (about the size of a good tangerine). If the gland is of greater size many urologists will opt for a retropubic prostatectomy, as the complications of a long TUR may be more than those of open operation. With a large gland in a frail patient, however, it is safer to resect as much as possible and then wait to see if he can void well: if he cannot, a further resection is performed. In modern urology units, retropubic prostatectomy has become a rare operation.

Complications

(a) *Of any prostatectomy*: The prostate is a very vascular organ so that some degree of postoperative haemorrhage is common. Careful attention to haemostasis at the end of the operation has made serious bleeding much less of a problem.

Lower urinary tract infection occurs in about 5 per cent of patients admitted as 'cold' cases. The incidence is higher in patients admitted with acute retention and catheterized for several days before surgery, and in patients with chronic retention with pre-existing infection. A completely closed catheter drainage system has considerably lessened this risk.

Incontinence following prostatectomy occurs in 2–3 per cent of cases, but in most it is transient. In the majority of permanent cases the cause is an inappropriate operation on a patient who had detrusor muscle instability without obstruction and whose operation has removed the critical amount of outflow resistance necessary for keeping the urine in. Occasionally even the most competent surgeon will damage the external sphincter and render the patient incontinent.

The bladder neck (or internal sphincter) is resected during prostatectomy, so that virtually all patients will have retrograde ejaculation. In a few patients with very small prostates, enough bladder neck function is retained to produce normal ejaculation. Reports vary about the effect of retrograde ejaculation on the enjoyment of sexual intercourse: it must depend to a certain extent on the patient's perception of the different phases of the act. In any event, it is essential that the patient be warned about this change before surgery. As a little seminal fluid leaks out in an antegrade fashion even with an incompetent bladder neck,

112 Disorders of bladder function

paternity is still possible (even though unlikely), and there have been a few embarrassing accidents!

Impotence after prostatectomy is uncommon, especially with transurethral resection. In patients whose libido is declining beforehand, any major illness or operation may mark the end of normal sexual activity. But for the sexually active man having intercourse perhaps 3 or 4 times a month, uncomplicated prostatectomy should make no difference.

There is so much 'barrack-room gossip' about the sexual consequences of surgery in general, and prostatectomy in particular, that it is incumbent on the surgeon to discuss the subject openly with the patient before the operation.

(b) *Of TUR*: The overwhelming advantage of TUR over retropubic prostatectomy is that there are few major complications. It is true that the technique is difficult to learn and, especially with large glands, tedious to perform, but these are not valid reasons for depriving the patient of so major a benefit.

The main early complication is absorption of irrigant fluid through the venous sinuses of the prostatic capsule. Almost all centres in England use isotonic glycine, so that absorption of small volumes is harmless. The glycine is metabolized and excreted from the kidneys as oxalate. If large volumes are absorbed, there is a severe dilutional effect which produces a specific syndrome of confusion (or even coma) and hyponatraemia. The volume alone may cause heart failure. The treatment is to discontinue intravenous and irrigant fluids and give diuretics. Most patients recover without sequelae, though death with cardiac arrest occurs occasionally.

(c) *Of retropubic prostatectomy*: This operation has all the complications that might be expected of a major abdominal operation. These include deep vein thrombosis, atelectasis with secondary chest infection and wound infection. The average hospital stay is about 9 days and convalescence about 6 weeks, compared with 5 days and 4 weeks respectively for TUR.

Results of removing obstruction

The only direct effect of removing obstruction is an increase in flow rate. After prostatectomy about 75 per cent of unstable detrusors will return to normal and a further 20 per cent will be improved. The more severe the unstable symptoms and the longer they have been present, the less likely is complete recovery. Return to normal functioning may take several months.

Chronic retention

The causes of this condition are set out above. It is one of the few 'obstructive' bladder lesions that can occur in women. The problem lies mainly with detrusor muscle failure, and the urethral resistance, especially in females, may be normal.

In males presenting with near-normal renal function and, particularly, normal haemoglobin level, there is no need to drain the bladder before prostatectomy. In renal failure with anaemia the bladder should be catheterized and surgery delayed until the renal function improves. All patients with chronic retention are likely to require a long period of catheterization after prostatectomy (often 6 or 8 weeks) before any measure of detrusor function returns.

In patients without a history of outflow obstruction – which includes virtually all females – urodynamic assessment is essential. If there is some residual detrusor function, reduction of outflow resistance by incision of the sphincters may be helpful. With very poor detrusor function ('low pressure, low flow') surgical treatment is unlikely to help. Detrusor function can be stimulated by parasympathomimetic drugs such as bethanecol, carbachol or distigmine bromide (given orally or parenterally) or by prostaglandin E2 instilled into the bladder. None of these drugs is very reliable and none has been subjected to large-scale scientific trial. Intermittent clean self-catheterization is probably the best long-term management of chronic retention, without obstruction.

Urethral stricture

Outflow obstruction may not always be due to prostatic enlargement. Urethral stricture, although less common than formerly, is still an important cause. The symptoms relate almost exclusively to the obstruction: poor stream and prolonged voiding. Unlike patients with BPH or bladder neck dyssynergia (see below), straining to void may improve the stream. Secondary effects on the bladder are uncommon, and although the detrusor may hypertrophy it seldom becomes unstable.

Aetiology

Any insult to the urethra may result in a circumferential fibrous stricture. In the developed world the commonest cause is trauma, usually iatrogenic. Any catheterization or instrumentation of the urethra may be followed by stricture at the areas of relative narrowing (close to the external meatus) or of curvature (the bulb). Ruptured urethra, complete or partial, almost always heals with stricture. World-wide, inadequately treated gonococcal urethritis is the commonest cause and the strictures are in the bulb.

Investigation

The diagnosis can usually be made on the history, perhaps supplemented by flow rate measurement. As the first line of treatment is endoscopic, suspected cases can reasonably be assessed by urethroscopy. If a complex stricture is suspected or open operation contemplated, a urethrogram is performed (see Chapter 2), but full visualization of the stricture is only possible with simultaneous antegrade and retrograde examination.

Management

The first line of treatment is endoscopic incision of the stricture under direct vision with an optical urethrotome. For about 50 per cent of patients a single urethrotomy, or urethrotomy repeated three or four times at intervals, will be curative.

For complicated strictures, especially those following a fractured pelvis and those not responding to urethrotomy, open urethral reconstruction is required. Many techniques are available, but all are complex, with a risk of recurrent stricture or fistula. For very short strictures excision and end-to-end anastomosis may be possible. For long strictures a suitable vascularized piece of skin is used to patch or completely replace the strictured segment.

Bladder neck dyssynergia

This most important condition is of comparatively recent discovery. Until the work of Turner-Warwick and colleagues in the early 1970s, anatomical bladder neck obstruction was diagnosed (probably far too often) on the cystoscopic appearances of the bladder neck. Dyssynergia, which does not have a visible effect on the bladder neck, went unrecognized.

In this condition, which is virtually confined to males, the bladder neck muscle fails to relax at the start of voiding. It does not actively contract, at least at the outset, and its resting pressure of 10–12 cm of water is maintained. In severe cases it may actively contract in response to increasing detrusor pressure.

The cause is unknown, and it is probably present from early childhood or even from birth. Obviously voiding is possible, and in the early stages the only symptom (if it can be called that) is a non-competitive stream – the boy who does not join in the games of peeing over the garden fence. In later life most patients develop a dislike of voiding in public. These symptoms must usually be especially asked for.

Eventually the detrusor, which is effectively being obstructed, develops unstable behaviour. It is at this stage that patients usually present and they are about 10–15 years younger than the average BPH patient. Symptoms may be accelerated by early prostatic enlargement, which is prevented, by the tight bladder neck, from expanding upwards into the bladder and so compresses the prostatic urethra from the start – the so-called 'trapped prostate'.

In the male the bladder neck fibres have an adrenergic innervation (see above). Although these patients do not have any recognizable autonomic neuropathy (except occasionally, when the condition occurs in diabetics) the symptoms are aggravated at times of generalized sympathetic activity. Conversely the alpha-adrenergic blocker phenoxybenzamine may improve the symptoms.

It is very important to distinguish these patients from those with benign prostatic hypertrophy. The definitive treatment is bladder neck incision at one site (usually 5 o'clock). The incidence of retrograde ejaculation is only 5–10 per cent thereafter. Prostatectomy is not required unless the prostate is also enlarged.

Although the bladder is trabeculated, there is no cystoscopic appearance on which the diagnosis can be made. In particular, the appearance of the bladder neck is irrelevant. Only video cystometrogram reveals the diagnosis.

Neuropathic lesions

The complex and finely balanced nature of urinary tract innervation makes it peculiarly susceptible to most neurological diseases. It is often the site of the first symptoms and, in conditions that recover, the last to get better. The care of the 'neuropathic bladder' has advanced so much in the last 40 years that it has become almost a specialty in its own right. Not the least of these advances is the realization that cutaneous diversion, far from being the solution to all problems, is merely the beginning of some new and major problems: even a very poor bladder is usually better than a conduit.

Other important considerations in long-term management include the general effects of the neurological process especially on manual dexterity, the effects of the bladder neuropathy on the kidneys, and the likelihood of the neurological condition changing (for better or worse). Renal failure is one of the commonest long-term complications of neurological disease, especially with spinal cord transection, from a variable combination of back pressure on the kidneys, chronic urinary infection and amyloidosis. The following sections give only a brief outline of the major bladder and urethral neuropathies.

Traumatic spinal cord transection

Whatever the level of transection, the immediate consequence is spinal shock in which all neural transmission below the lesion stops. The bladder goes into retention. Mismanagement at this stage will sow the seeds of intractable long-term complications: the introduction of infection is the most serious. Patients are best managed by intermittent catheterization using a small catheter and meticulous aseptic technique. An indwelling catheter will nearly always cause infection.

With time, reflex detrusor and sphincter activity gradually returns. It may take several months before a stable state is reached. The function of the urinary tract muscle depends on the level and completeness of the lesion. As the centre for coordination between detrusor and sphincter is in the pons, all spinal cord lesions will involve imbalance between these two sets of muscles.

High lesions, down to the mid-thoracic segments, cause the detrusor to contract at high pressure. The external sphincter and periurethral muscles are spastic so that voiding is usually impossible. Reflex voiding can be initiated by stroking or massaging the lower abdomen (Crede manoeuvre). In some cases 'spontaneous' voiding occurs at the end of the detrusor contractions when the periurethral muscles relax.

Vesicoureteric reflux quickly develops, so that the full force of detrusor pressure during storage and attempted voiding is transmitted to the kidneys. Renal failure in males is inevitable unless the external sphincter is incised to lessen the pressure. Females seldom have serious upper tract damage from back pressure alone.

With low thoracic and high lumbar lesions the reflex detrusor activity is at lower pressure and poorly sustained. Although the sphincters are at lower pressure, voiding is incomplete and progressive chronic retention develops. Contractions leave a large residual. Patients usually have intermittent dribbling incontinence. Upper tract dilatation, compounded by chronic infection, leads to renal failure unless the outflow resistance is reduced.

In lesions of the conus medullaris at the bottom of the spinal cord and of the corda equina, the detrusor, sphincter and pelvic floor are flaccid. Voiding can be accomplished by a combination of the Crede manoeuvre and abdominal straining, though this often leaves a residual. Incontinence of the stress type is usual.

With the lower lesions it is often possible for patients to manage themselves by clean intermittent self-catheterization. The pressure and the residual are thus kept low enough to prevent upper tract damage. If the functional capacity of the bladder before incontinence is high enough, this technique maintains continence.

Lesions of the brain

Lesions of the brain frequently carry a poor prognosis which affects attitudes to the urinary problems that accompany them. This does not lessen the requirement for good management, because even a brief period of incontinence is very distressing; but it does mean that techniques that would not normally be contemplated for use over many years can be brought in. Such central lesions usually produce impairment of manual dexterity, weakness and sometimes confusion which further complicate management.

Strokes

Strokes have a variable effect on the bladder. The detrusor becomes unstable, leading to urgency and urge incontinence. Patients may have sufficient control that a bottle or commode placed close at hand allows continence; otherwise a condom appliance or indwelling catheter is the best management. Anticholinergic agents such as probanthine or emepromium are sometimes effective in reducing instability and increasing functional capacity, but side-effects in the elderly are often severe.

Parkinson's disease

Bladder dysfunction occurs in about 70 per cent of patients with Parkinson's disease, and the problems are certainly aggravated by stiffness and immobility. About two-thirds of affected patients have detrusor instability which is improved by the anticholinergic drugs normally given for Parkinson's disease. Urethral function is usually normal, and L-Dopa, which has an alpha-adrenergic effect, may cause retention but does not help the detrusor to become stable.

The other third have detrusor hypotonia which is obviously worsened by all anti-Parkinsonian drugs. Intermittent self-catheterization is unlikely to be successful as urethral sensation is normal and manual dexterity poor. Outflow resistance can be reduced by prostatectomy (or sphincterotomy in females), but if the bladder still cannot be emptied, an indwelling catheter is necessary.

In all elderly males with central neurological lesions and bladder symptoms, the possibility of prostatic obstruction must be considered. Urodynamic assessment will often indicate obstruction but cannot predict which patients will respond to its relief. There is a good chance of making the patient incontinent, and this risk weighs heavily when contemplating surgery.

Peripheral neuropathies and demyelinating diseases

The commonest diseases in this group are the Guillain-Barré syndrome and multiple sclerosis. The urinary tract is affected at some stage in virtually all cases. The nature of functional disturbance depends on the nerves affected, is variable and may recover. Management must, therefore, be very conservative as that which is right for the patient this year may be wrong next year.

The nature of these conditions requires repeated urodynamic evaluations which should include urethral pressure profiles. Fortunately, the denervation is rarely complete and the effects are therefore milder than those seen with spinal cord transections. Renal damage is uncommon. Management is along the lines set out for spinal cord injuries.

Incontinence

Urinary incontinence, whatever the underlying cause, is a most distressing symptom. Although it is not itself dangerous except in patients already at risk from bed sores, it can completely destroy a patient's enjoyment of life. Self-confidence is lost and social life stops. Patients find it a difficult subject to discuss with their doctor and impossible with their friends. In severe cases keeping clean and dry becomes a whole-time occupation unless proper management is set up. It is far more common than is generally believed, largely because of the unwillingness of subjects to present themselves. In some degree it may affect up to 4 per cent of the population.

The earlier parts of the chapter have already indicated many of the principal causes of incontinence. In most cases careful history and examination should identify a cause, and sophisticated tests such as urodynamics are not always needed. Unfortunately, incontinence is one of the subjects on which many patients are often unable to give a coherent history.

Congenital anomalies

Several of the anomalies described in Chapter 12 cause incontinence. Some are obvious and the incontinence is but a side issue in the overall management. A few are very subtle, but they are rewarding to find as treatment is usually successful.

The upper ureter of a duplex kidney may open distal to the sphincters. The bladder will fill and empty normally, but the child is, nonetheless, always wet. This classical history demands meticulous investigation as the ectopic opening is very difficult to find and the upper renal moiety may not concentrate radiological contrast. Fortunately, the ureter is usually dilated and is seen on ultrasound.

Nocturnal enuresis

Children normally become dry by day at between 2 and 3 years old, and at night by 5 years old. Those who wet the bed beyond this age are enuretic and require treatment.

The simple enuretic has no daytime symptoms, although the functional capacity is less than in age-matched controls. At night the pattern is variable, some wetting every night, some 3-4 nights per week, and some having periods of several weeks when there is no wetting at all. This history is very important as simple enuretics require no special investigation and, in 95 per cent of cases, will become dry by 15 years old at the latest.

It is commoner in boys than girls and there is a high familial incidence. The aetiology is unknown, but a developmental defect must play some part as it usually gets better with time and primary enuresis beginning in adult life is almost unknown. Although many cases appear to be precipitated by an upset - such as divorce, moving house or changing schools - there is no evidence that it is primarily a psychiatric condition. Patients have no identifiable anatomical, neurological or psychiatric anomaly.

Although the prognosis is good, treatment is still required to save social embarrassment for the child and years of sheet washing for the parent. Most cases respond to a regimen of potting at the parents' bed-time and an anticholinergic. In practice the most useful anticholinergics are the tricyclic antidepressants imipramine (25 mg) or tryptizol (10 mg) nocte. Overdosage has serious or even lethal consequences, and parents must be instructed to keep the drugs locked up. For children over 7 or 8 years, conditioning by an alarm that rings loudly when the first drop of urine appears is the treatment of choice.

Detrusor instability

The detrusor may become unstable from any of the obstructive or neurological causes already discussed. When the detrusor pressure exceeds the urethral closure pressure the urine leaks out. Symptomatically, the complaint is of frequency and inability to get to the lavatory in time - urge incontinence.

Unfortunately, no drug specifically inhibits detrusor contractions. The anticholinergic drugs used have several unwanted effects, including a dry mouth and constipation. Furthermore, even with complete cholinergic blockade by atropine, the detrusor can still contract to some extent. Probanthine (15-30mg four-hourly) is probably the most effective. Emepronium bromide (Cetiprin) (200 mg six-hourly) is the most popular agent, even though double-blind trials have failed to show much advantage over placebo. Gastrointestinal absorption is variable, which further complicates its use.

The most promising agent in recent trials has been Oxybutinine (5 mg t.d.s.). Its exact mode of action is uncertain: it is, *in vitro*, a smooth-muscle relaxant but also has local anaesthetic and anticholinergic activity. Several other drugs are under trial at present.

For severe instability the possibility of surgery exists. Bladder distension is relatively simple and widely used, though of limited value. Under epidural anaesthetic a balloon (e.g. Helmstein's balloon) is put into the bladder and filled with water. The intravesical pressure is maintained mid-way between diastolic and systolic blood pressure for six hours. The procedure may be complicated by bladder rupture. Even in those patients who respond the benefit is short-lived and the procedure has to be repeated. Progressive reduction in real bladder capacity and decreased compliance are long-term complications.

More invasive surgical procedures must be reserved for the few cases whose incontinence is truly disabling, who have failed to respond to adequate trials of non-surgical treatment and have been fully assessed. The operations are major and therefore have major complications; their success is unpredictable, especially outside the units that have popularized them.

For patients with a normal bladder capacity under anaesthetic (450 ml or more) some form of denervation is best. Sacral neurectomy or transection of the full thickness of the bladder wall just above the trigone are the most successful. If the capacity is small, the bladder, except for the trigone, is removed and replaced by caecum or colon.

In primary instability and in some secondary instability, central control of bladder function is not completely lost. Thus retraining – re-establishing control by the cerebral cortex – is feasible and in some hands highly successful. It requires a well-motivated patient who is able to understand the nature of the problem. The simplest method involves teaching the patient to increase gradually the voiding interval and to resist the desire to void. More complex methods include biofeedback techniques and hypnotism. Unfortunately, all these methods require a good deal of medical time and so have not gained general acceptance.

Sphincter incompetence

Even though the normal bladder pressure is low, the urethral sphincters, especially in women, may be rendered incompetent by quite minor damage. In men, isolated sphincter damage is nearly always due to trauma, either accidental with a fractured pelvis or surgical. In women it is usually due to displacement or distortion of the urethra from prolapse.

If the sphincters are totally non-functioning the patient has continuous dribbling incontinence. Partial function allows some storage, but there is leakage or uncontrolled voiding with any rise in intra-abdominal or intravesical pressure – so-called 'stress incontinence'. Clearly the amount of stress required to produce incontinence is proportional to the residual sphincter function. In women with prolapse it may be only sudden, explosive rises in pressure (such as occur with sneezing and coughing) that produce leakage. In men whose sphincters have been ablated by injudicious prostatectomy, storage may only occur when asleep in bed, any movement producing uncontrolled bladder emptying.

Unfortunately, the history is not totally diagnostic because such stress may provoke unstable detrusor contractions. Furthermore, women especially may develop a habit of frequent voiding on the principle that 'that which goes down the lavatory cannot come out in the knickers'. In doubtful cases (which includes all cases of post-prostatectomy incontinence) urodynamic studies must be done. About 5 per cent of otherwise normal young women have some degree of stress incontinence. After each succeeding pregnancy the incidence rises owing to damage to the periurethral ligaments and muscles. As prolapse carries the urethra and its sphincters out of the abdominal cavity, intra-abdominal pressure is expended more on the bladder and fails to help the urethra to stay closed. Furthermore, the urethra moves further from the symphysis and loses its acute angle with the bladder base, so intra-abdominal pressure has even less chance of keeping it closed. The atrophy of the pelvic ligaments that follows the menopause worsens the prolapse.

The young women with life-long stress incontinence probably have a congenital weakness of the sphincter. It sometimes improves with the menarche or with administration of the contraceptive pill. Otherwise surgery is required.

Better care of patients during pregnancy and labour has lowered the incidence of prolapse. It still remains a common problem in gynaecology clinics. There is no really useful drug therapy, though the alpha-adrenergic agonist phenylpropanolamine (50 mg t.d.s.) may help some mild cases. The synthetic amphetamine mazindol (1 or 2 mg daily) has produced same impressive results, though the mode of action is unknown. Both drugs have unpleasant side-effects and are unsuitable for elderly patients with cardiovascular disease.

Surgery is primarily undertaken by the gynaecologist. For the majority of cases, repositioning of the bladder neck, urethra and, if necessary, the uterus from a vaginal approach is satisfactory. For recurrent cases, congenital problems and those with a stenosed vagina, open operation is required. Bladder neck and urethral repositioning (Marshall–Marchetti–Krantz repair), provision of a bladder neck sling or, in extreme cases, tightening of the bladder neck, all have their advocates.

In men, total destruction of sphincters is the rule. A few sub-total cases will respond to the same drug regimens as outlined for women. For the remainder, the otherwise hopeless outlook has been revolutionized by the introduction of the artificial sphincter. Unfortunately, they are expensive, prone to infection and to mechanical failure, but are entirely justified when simpler methods have failed.

Urinary diversion

Great ingenuity has gone into the devising of alternative methods of storing and eliminating urine. All of them have major long-term complications. Following cystectomy for cancer, some form of diversion is clearly essential. Aside from this absolute indication, diversion is the resort of the urologically destitute. Almost any bladder is better than diversion.

Ileal conduit and colon conduit

Diversion of urine into an intestinal conduit has been the method of choice for over 30 years. The ureters are anastomosed to the proximal end of an isolated ileal or colonic segment, and the distal end forms a cutaneous stoma which empties into a bag adherent to the skin (Fig. 11.2). The advantage of colon over ileum is that it has sufficient muscle to allow an antireflux anastomosis with the ureters.

Conduits work very well in the short term. However, the intestine generates a high pressure which is worsened by the stomal stenosis that occurs in at least 50 per cent of cases. The stenosis also leads to stasis, a high resting volume in the conduit, and thus to infection. The combination of infection and high pressure leads to damage to 50–75 per cent of kidneys at 15 years. The long-term results

Urinary diversion 121

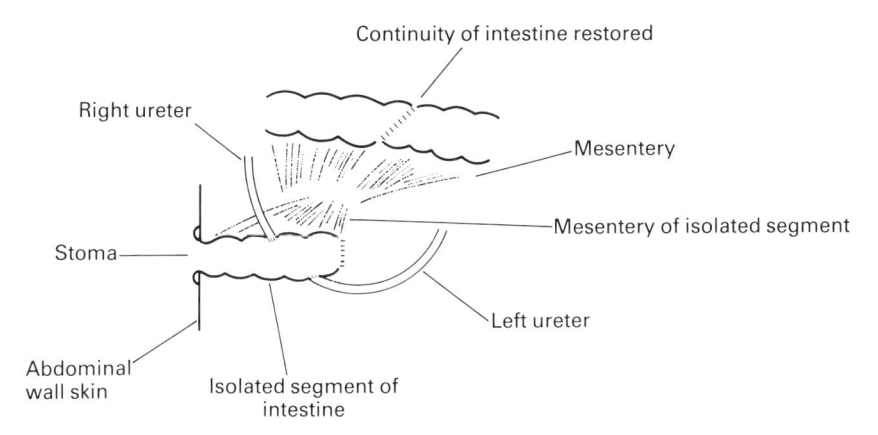

Fig. 11.2 Urinary diversion by intestinal conduit.

of colon conduit with successful antireflux anastomosis may prove to be rather better.

Ureterosigmoidostomy

The diversion of urine into the faecal stream for subsequent evacuation per rectum is theoretically an excellent idea, especially as no cutaneous bag is required. The technique has been thoroughly refined over the 100 years or so that it has been practised.

The early complications have been largely controlled. Ascending infection occurs less often with the use of an antireflux anastomosis with the ureters, and antibiotics have lessened its effects on the kidneys.

The physiological response of the sigmoid to the presence of acidic urine in the lumen is to secrete bicarbonate and absorb chloride. The resulting metabolic hyperchloraemic acidosis if untreated is eventually fatal. However, proper electrolyte supplement with oral bicarbonate has largely eliminated this problem.

Other minor problems include the inadequacy of the anal sphincter (unless the operation is done in early childhood), and the very unpleasant smell of the rectal effluent.

In the long-term, damage still occurs in about 50 per cent of kidneys at 15 years. More serious, however, is the long-term risk of adenocarcinoma precisely at the anastomosis between ureter and sigmoid. As patients survive longer the risk is becoming more apparent, and it is at least 100 times the risk of colonic carcinoma occurring in the ordinary population. The risk begins after 15 years, with a mean time of 23 years. At least 10 per cent of ureterosigmoidostomy patients will develop carcinoma even if the urine and faeces are mixed for only a few months and the urine is subsequently diverted elsewhere. The only protection is excision of the lower ureter with a generous cuff of colon.

Continent conduits

Dissatisfaction with external devices has provoked a search for some method of making a continent intestinal reservoir. Until recently success has been limited, but the Kock technique will probably prove a breakthrough. Sufficient length of ileum is isolated and used to make a pouch to which the ureters are anastomosed. The outlet is controlled by a short length of intussuscepted ileum which acts as a non-return valve. The pouch is emptied by self-catheterization.

12
Congenital anomalies

The genitourinary system is the commonest site of congenital anomalies. The majority are apparent at birth, though there is a steady rate of presentation throughout life of lesions producing little change in organ function.

In fetal life renal lesions severe enough to cause renal failure produce oligohydramnios and are apparent in pregnancy. The present practice of regular uterine ultrasound examinations in pregnancy is identifying some dilated urinary tracts in fetuses: at present the usefulness of these findings is confined to ensuring swift management after birth, but they lay the way for intrauterine intervention when the science has developed sufficiently.

Renal anomalies

Anomalies of blood supply

The kidneys develop from the mesonephros on the posterior wall of the coelomic cavity. Although the blood supply is initially from several vessels, all but one artery and vein on each side disappear by the time of full renal development in 80 per cent of people. Twenty per cent will have extra or aberrant vessels which must be searched for during nephrectomy; the incidence is higher with renal parenchymal anomalies.

Anomalies of parenchymal development

Single renal cysts are extremely common and are of no importance. They are usually an incidental finding during urological investigation and may be briefly mistaken for carcinomas until defined by renal ultrasound. Malignant change rarely, if ever, occurs. They may be aspirated if there is a diagnostic doubt, but otherwise no treatment is needed.

Multiple cysts occur in several distinct forms. They usually cause sufficient disruption of the parenchyma to produce renal failure. In the rare condition of infantile multicystic kidneys, usually bilateral, there is so little functioning parenchyma that oligohydramnios is present. Infants born alive develop renal failure early. The treatment is as for end-stage renal failure (see Chapter 4), but is complicated by the young age. Other congenital anomalies are common and early death is usual.

Adult polycystic disease is an autosomal dominant condition. Patients present in the 4th decade of life with large, often huge, multicystic kidneys and renal failure. There is an increased incidence of cysts in unaffected family members with normal renal function.

Aside from the renal failure, the complications of the cysts may require treatment. Haemorrhage, infection and pain are common. If it is possible to identify a single offending cyst, it can be aspirated: obviously this is difficult and nephrectomy may be necessary. However, polycystic kidneys usually continue to produce erythropoietin and several hundred millilitres of dilute urine until very late in the course of the disease; for this reason, renal failure is easier to endure and nephrectomy should be a last resort.

The kidney may fail to develop altogether (aplasia) or may develop in such a rudimentary form that it has no useful function (dysplasia). Aplasia is associated with absent ureter and hemitrigone. Dysplasia is often associated with vesicoureteric reflux: indeed it may be that severe intrauterine reflux caused the dysplasia. Unilateral anomalies present as chance findings, while the very rare bilateral anomalies usually result in intrauterine death.

Anomalies of position

The commonest anomaly of position is the 'horseshoe': the kidneys are rotated so that the pelves lie anteriorly and the lower poles are fused in the mid-line (very rarely the upper poles or even all four poles are fused). The ureters lie anteriorly and there are multiple, segmental arteries and veins (Fig. 12.1).

The horseshoe kidney is sometimes associated with unilateral or bilateral pelviureteric junction obstruction. There is a slightly increased risk of renal adenocarcinoma. The rotated position of the kidneys may obscure the calyceal distortion of a small carcinoma. Surgery is difficult because of the multiplicity of large vessels, and division of the isthmus between the two sides is particularly bloody.

Very rarely kidneys may be ectopic in the bony pelvis or may lie on the opposite side (crossed ectopia, Fig. 12.2). The ureters enter the bladder in the correct position.

Renal pelvic and ureteric anomalies

Pelviureteric junction obstruction

In infancy, unilateral PUJ obstruction presents with unexplained abdominal pain or with haematuria after a trivial injury. Urinary tract infection from PUJ obstruction alone is rare and should always promote a search for another anomaly, particularly vesicoureteric reflux. Bilateral PUJ obstruction may present similarly or with renal failure.

Uncomplicated PUJ obstruction is managed by the principles outlined in Chapter 10. If vesicoureteric reflux is also present, it should be treated first (vide infra). The PUJ obstruction may be secondary to reflux and may not require

Renal pelvic and ureteric anomalies 125

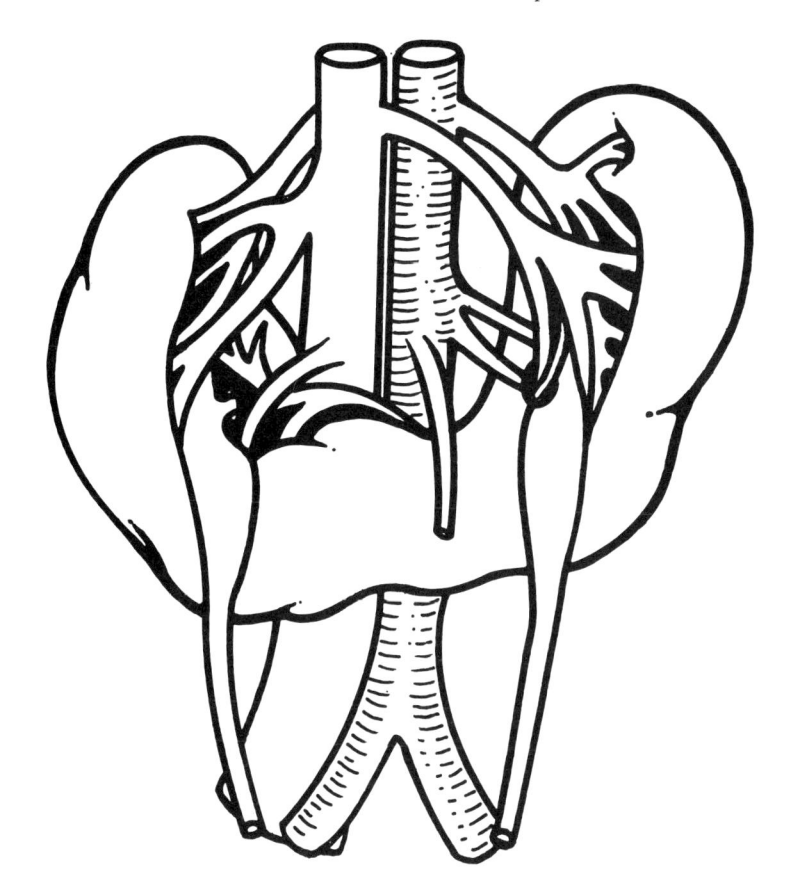

Fig. 12.1 Anterior view of a horseshoe kidney.

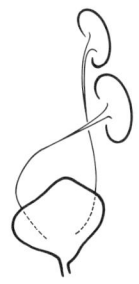

Fig. 12.2 Crossed renal ectopia.

surgery when the reflux has been corrected. Both ends of a ureter should not be operated on at the same time, especially in the infant, as the ureter may be devascularized.

126 *Congenital anomalies*

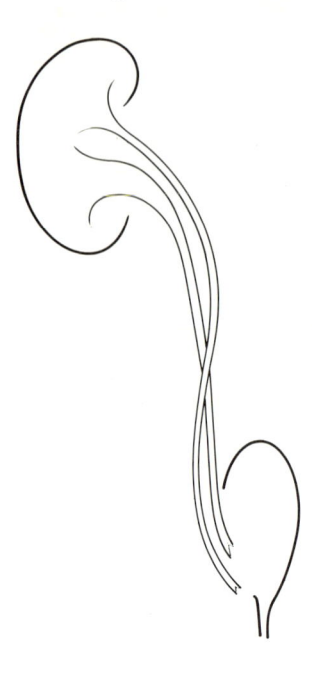

Fig. 12.3 Duplication of the right ureter.

Duplicated ureter

In its simplest form only the renal pelvis is duplicated and in full form duplication is complete down to the bladder. When there are two ureters they always cross, so that the ureter from the upper pole of the kidney enters the bladder below that from the lower pole (Fig. 12.3).

When there are no complications this anomaly is inconsequential. However, the following are the commonest complications.

Vesicoureteric reflux into the lower pole ureter

Commonly the renal lower pole will have been so damaged by the time of presentation that heminephrectomy and ureterectomy is the best management. Occasionally more conservative surgical or even medical treatment is possible (see p. 127). As both ureters run in the same sheath the unaffected one will often have to be reimplanted in the bladder, whatever is done to the affected one.

Ectopia of the upper pole ureter

The ureter may open anywhere on the line from the normal position in the bladder to the proximal urethra. It may also open directly on to the perineum or in the vagina. Ectopia is much commoner in girls. If the opening is on or below the bladder neck it usually produces a specific form of incontinence (see Chapter 11).

If the history is suggestive, search for the duplicity must be exhaustive, including ultrasound, isotope renal scintigraphy and examination under anaesthetic. When found, the upper pole of the kidney and its ureter are removed. Great care must be taken at the lower end as the ureter passes close to or through the muscle of the bladder neck.

Ureterocele of upper pole ureter

The mucosa of the lower end of the ureter may fail to develop an adequate orifice so that the system is obstructed. The tiny opening that is present is commonly ectopic and is sometimes below the bladder neck, resulting in incontinence. The mucosa balloons out and is seen as a filling defect in the bladder on IVU: the shape is characteristic and resembles a cobra's head. Recurrent infection is the commonest presentation in those who are not incontinent. Ureterocele may also occur in a non-duplex ureter (Fig. 12.4).

Simple incision of the ureterocele is seldom satisfactory, both because the upper pole is dilated and has poor function, and because the incision produces vesicoureteric reflux. Partial nephrectomy, ureterectomy and ureterocelectomy is usually necessary.

Vesicoureteric reflux

This is the single most important congenital anomaly of the urinary system. Normally each ureter runs obliquely through the bladder muscle and has a long submucosal tunnel which prevents reflux of urine from the bladder at any stage in the cycle of filling and emptying. If this valve is incompetent reflux occurs during voiding or, in severe cases, even during the phase of bladder filling.

The natural history of vesicoureteric reflux is a matter of dispute. It is found in 50 per cent of children with recurrent urinary infection, more often in girls than boys. In most it is present at birth, but in some it only occurs when the bladder urine is infected.

The incompetent vesicoureteric valve allows the bladder pressure to act directly on the ureter and kidney. If the reflux occurs only during voiding the back pressure causes little dilatation. Continuous reflux during storage and voiding phases results in hydronephrosis and atrophy of the renal parenchyma. However, in children with normal bladders the intravesical pressure is low, and back-pressure effects may not be very important. Reflux occurring with conditions causing high intravesical pressure (such as neuropathy and outflow obstruction) causes severe renal damage.

Reflux is commonly associated with recurrent bacterial cystitis or asymptomatic bacteriuria. The consequences of infection with reflux are disputed. There is no doubt that infection perpetuates reflux, and successful control of infection is followed by resolution of reflux in nearly 80 per cent of patients between 6 and 15 years of age.

Infection is associated with segmental renal damage in some cases, usually of the upper or lower poles – so-called 'reflux nephropathy'. On IVU the calyces

128 *Congenital anomalies*

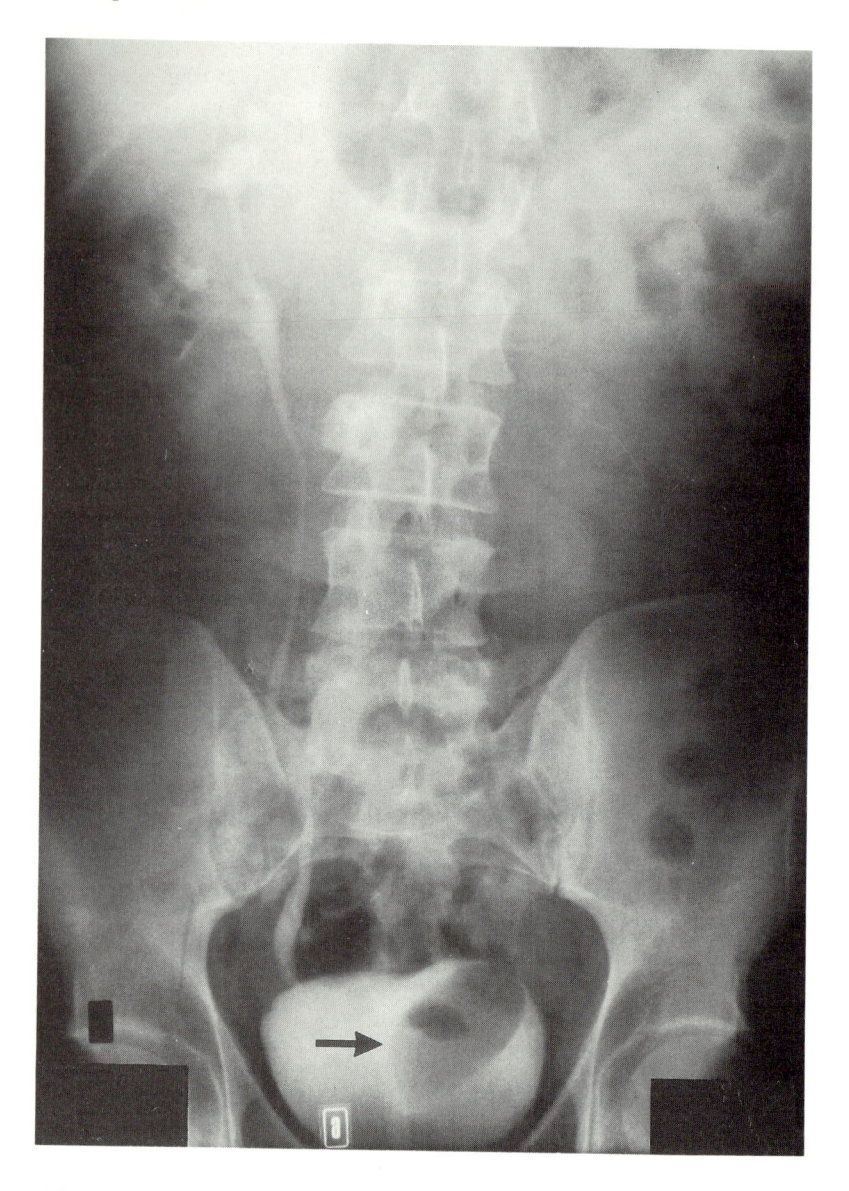

Fig. 12.4 IVU: The right kidney and ureter are normal. On the left there is no function. In the bladder there is a smooth filling defect on the left characteristic of a ureterocele.

are deformed and the overlying parenchyma is scarred with indentation of the renal outline. The damage was thought to be due to chronic pyelonephritis, but current research suggests a different answer. It is most likely that some kidneys have abnormal renal papillae, especially at the upper and lower poles, that allow intrarenal reflux. The renal damage from infected reflux can only occur in these areas. The first episode of acute pyelonephritis appears to destroy the renal parenchyma within a few days, and further episodes of infection probably cause no further damage. This 'big bang' theory explains the curious distribution of scars, often affecting only one kidney when both are exposed to vesicoureteric reflux, and the patchy and non-progressive course in affected kidneys.

After 5 or 6 years of age the abnormal papillae have matured and intrarenal reflux usually disappears. Thus children who have escaped any urinary infection until this age are unlikely to develop scars even if they do subsequently get an infection.

Severe bilateral reflux can cause renal failure which may not be prevented by correction of the reflux. Even minor areas of scarring need careful follow-up as there is a 10-20 per cent incidence of hypertension in adolescence or early adult life. In later life continued reflux may predispose to lower urinary tract infection, but it seldom causes renal damage except during pregnancy or when bladder outflow obstruction occurs (as in men with prostatic enlargement). Late renal damage causing renal failure can occur, and persistent refluxers need careful follow-up.

Management

Children, especially those less than 6 years old, with suspected urinary infection must be promptly treated and investigated. There is no virtue in waiting for a second infection to occur as 75 per cent of children having one UTI will have a second one anyway, and the price of investigating the extra 25 per cent is the saving of some children from renal damage.

Immediately the child is seen a mid-stream or clean catch urine must be collected for microscopy and culture. In infants urine is collected in a self-adhesive sterile bag enclosing the genitalia. Treatment should be started at once (without waiting for the culture result) with a broad-spectrum antibiotic active against Gram-negative organisms, such as trimethoprim or ampicillin.

The ideal programme of investigation for children presenting with urinary infection is a plain X-ray for stones, urinary tract ultrasound with the bladder full and empty, and micturating cystourethrogram. Further investigation may follow, depending on the abnormalities detected by this screen.

Patients with reflux require treatment for the reflux and for recurrent infections – the two may not be the same.

For infection the first line of treatment is with antibiotics. Infants with reflux who are diagnosed before renal damage has occurred are kept on continuous antibiotics at least until they are 6 years old. In older children, and especially in those who have already acquired renal scars, it is reasonable to give antibiotics only for episodes of proven infection with symptoms: the mere presence of bacteriuria does not cause any damage. In this group, continuous antibiotics are reserved for patients with frequently recurrent episodes of cystitis. Eighty per cent of refluxing ureters will stop refluxing spontaneously when the urine is continuously sterile.

The surgical treatment for reflux consists of reimplantation of the ureter in a new submucosal tunnel in the bladder which prevents reflux. Cure of reflux is possible in about 90 per cent of uncomplicated cases, but about 5 per cent of successfully reimplanted ureters subsequently develop stenosis.

The indications for reimplantation are controversial, but even amongst the enthusiasts for surgery the operation has become less common than it was around 1980. The main indication is failure of conservative management to cure reflux or to control infection. If infection is controlled and reflux persists, a very good case can be made for ignoring the reflux: however, many paediatric surgeons are reluctant to allow children, especially girls, to grow beyond their care with persistent reflux.

A major area of conflict exists in the management of infants with reflux but no nephropathy. Important trials are under way at present to compare reimplantation with continuous antibiotics: preliminary results show no advantage of one over the other in terms of renal preservation.

Grossly refluxing ureters draining poorly functioning kidneys should not be reimplanted. It does not improve renal function. Dilated ureters have poor propulsive function and reimplantation may produce resistance to flow sufficient to obstruct the kidney; function may thus be worsened.

Congenital megaureter

It is tempting to believe that dilatation of the urinary tract is a consequence of obstruction. Clearly a refluxing ureter, described above, is not obstructed (though occasional examples are seen of ureters that are both refluxing and obstructed). The relationship of obstruction to dilatation is dealt with in Chapter 10.

The congenital megaureter is a curious condition. Minor forms, fusiform dilatations of the lower ureter, are common chance findings at all ages. In the grossest form the whole upper tract is dilated with much loss of renal parenchyma. Anything in between is possible.

In some cases there is a physiological obstruction at the ureterovesical junction analogous to that found at the pelviureteric junction. For these reimplantation with reduction of the ureter is indicated.

In a great many cases no obstruction is found. As recurrent infection is the commonest presentation, conservative treatment is indicated, reserving surgery for failed medical treatment or where renal scintigraphy provides evidence of progressive renal damage.

Vary rarely megaureter occurs as part of a general abnormality of urinary tract development.

Bladder anomalies

Physiological abnormalities of bladder storage, control and emptying are common, especially in association with neurological anomalies. They are covered in Chapter 11. Anatomical anomalies are rare and are beyond the scope of this book.

Urethral anomalies

Posterior urethral valves

In the male urethra, congenital mucosal folds of various shapes may occur. Characteristically they impede the outward flow of urine, but not the inward passage of a catheter. Although uncommon, posterior urethral valves are a very important source of urological morbidity in boys.

Valves cause a poor urinary stream which may be obvious soon after birth. The detrusor muscle becomes hypertrophied. The upper tracts may become secondarily dilated with back-pressure atrophy of the kidneys due to vesicoureteric reflux or obstruction. The characteristically dilated urinary tract may be seen on uterine ultrasound examination before birth. Late presentation in childhood may be with renal failure, recurrent infection or chance finding of an enlarged bladder.

A micturating cystourethrogram confirms the diagnosis. The bladder is thick-walled. There may be reflux. The prostatic urethra is dilated down to the site of the valves (Fig. 12.5).

Surgical treatment consists of incision of the valves transurethrally. It is seldom necessary to resect them; this is fortunate as the procedure carries a high risk of incontinence from external sphincter damage.

Following treatment most cases develop normal bladder function. Unfortunately, the high intravesical pressure that precedes valve surgery has nearly always caused renal damage. By early adult life about 25 per cent of patients have raised serum creatinine, and a further 25 per cent are in end-stage renal failure.

Hypospadias

The male anterior urethra forms as an open plate on the ventrum of the penis. The lateral edges of the urethral plate close together to form a tube. The closure proceeds from proximal to distal and is complete by the 14th week of fetal life. If the urethra fails to close completely, the external urethral meatus is left in a proximal position: the condition is known as hypospadias. Minor degrees with the meatus lying in or just proximal to the coronal sulcus are common. Severe degrees with the meatus in the mid shaft or at the penoscrotal junction are rare (Fig. 12.6).

Hypospadias is always associated with an incomplete prepuce which is deficient ventrally. Shaft and proximal hypospadias is associated with ventral curvature on erection known as chordee. There is seldom any association with other congenital lesions except when the meatus is very proximal.

Boys born with hypospadias must not be circumcised. Construction of a urethra should be performed, usually with prepucial skin. At the same time the subcutaneous fibrous tissue that causes chordee is excised. The timing of surgery is controversial: traditionally it was delayed until the infant was out of nappies, but many paediatric urologists now prefer to operate when the child is 1 year old. Surgery should always be completed before school attendance starts.

132 Congenital anomalies

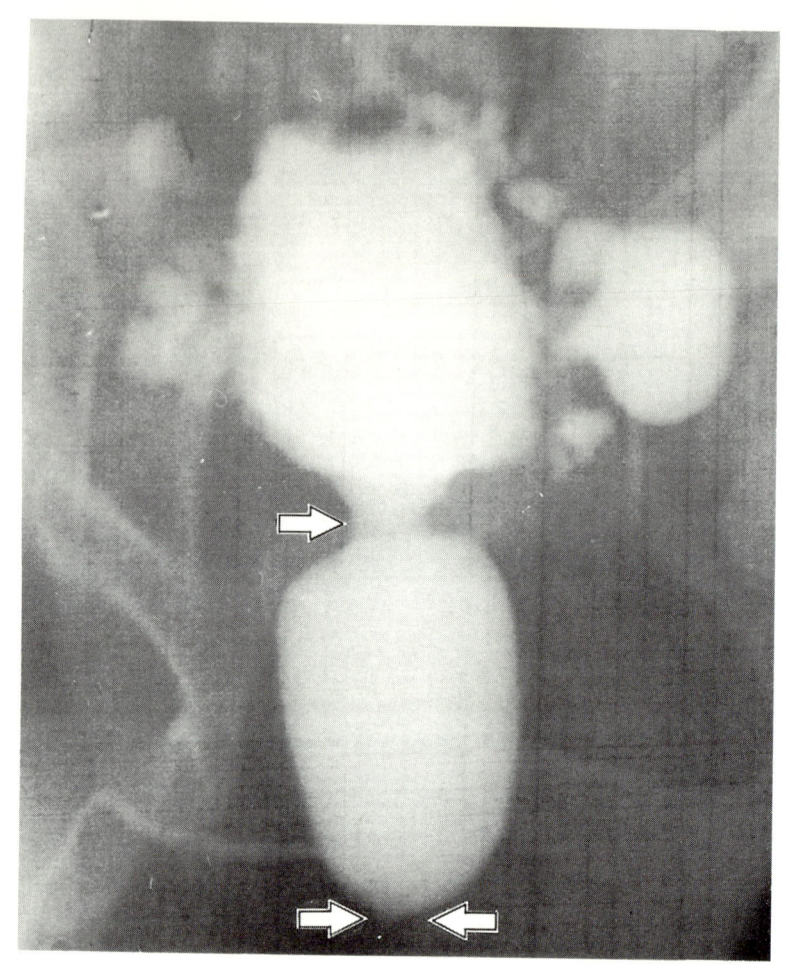

Fig. 12.5 Cystogram of a patient with posterior urethral valves, showing a small irregular bladder with diverticula and a widely dilated, smooth prostatic urethra (bladder neck: one arrow; valve site: two arrows).

The testes

Undescended testes (cryptorchism)

In normal early fetal life the gonad lies on the dorsal wall of the coelomic cavity caudal to the kidney. By the sixth week of fetal life in the male it is fixed in position by the gubernaculum. Normal descent occurs partly by cranial growth of the lumbar area and partly by the activity of the gubernaculum. The gubernaculum initially grows in diameter and widens the inguinal canal. Then, under the influence of dihydrotestosterone, the gubernaculum degenerates. A

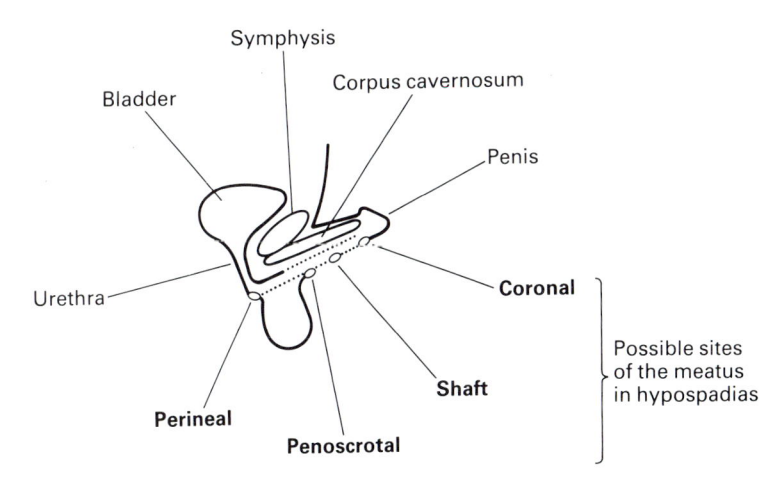

Fig. 12.6 Types of hypospadias.

combination of gubernacular degeneration and raised intra-abdominal pressure forces the testes, fairly rapidly, into the scrotum. Descent is completed by the 8th month *in utero*.

Undescended testes were first described, like so many other things, by John Hunter (1762). Strictly speaking there are two varieties: ectopic testes which are rare, where the testes lie outside the normal path of descent (e.g. in the anterior abdominal wall); and maldescended, the usual problem, where the testes are in the normal path of descent, but have failed to reach the scrotum. Management in each case is the same.

Maldescent testes must be distinguished from retractile testes. With the latter the cremaster is overactive, so pulling the testicle out of the scrotum, especially in the cold or during periods of anxiety. Retractile testes do not require treatment.

If there is a single cause of cryptorchism it is unknown, though there are many theories. In the majority of cases, the lesion occurs in isolation with no other anomalies, and it is likely that there is a primary abnormality in the testis itself. In a few cases it is associated with endocrine or chromosomal anomalies, so that both sides are nearly always undescended.

Unilateral or bilateral undescended testes are found in about 3 per cent of full-term, and about 30 per cent of premature, male infants. Descent in the first three months of life does occur, but thereafter spontaneous descent is uncommon. About 2.5 per cent of army recruits are found to have cryptorchism.

Long-term consequences of cryptorchism

(a) *Fertility:* It is uncertain how many unilateral or bilateral cryptorchid boys are subsequently infertile. Long-term studies are lacking and the age at which corrective surgery is performed may be critical. Bilateral cryptorchism, uncorrected, virtually always causes azoospermia. In the first year of life, there are no histological differences between undescended and normal testes, even with electron microscopy. Thereafter progressively more marked changes are seen in the undescended testis. Ultimately the tubules are replaced by collagen. About 30 per cent of unilateral cases and 60 per cent of bilateral cases successfully corrected in mid-childhood are infertile.

(b) *Malignancy:* Boys with cryptorchism are about 35 times more likely to develop germ cell tumours than normals. The higher the testis, the greater the risk. In unilateral cases the risk is also increased on the normally descended side, though less so than on the descended side. Successful correction does not remove the risk.

Management

In examining the boy it is important to have a warm room, warm hands and a warm approach, otherwise even the most normal testes may disappear into the neck of the scrotum. With gentle manipulation, retractile testes can be brought into the scrotum. If there are other anomalies present, the possibility of chromosome or endocrine anomalies must be considered. Bilateral cryptorchism associated with any disturbance of urinary function suggests the rare diagnosis of *prune belly syndrome*. This syndrome consists of cryptorchism, bizarre urinary tract anomalies and variable absence of the anterior abdominal muscles. The absent muscle gives the abdominal wall a wrinkled appearance similar to the skin of a prune.

Traditionally, treatment is undertaken when subjects are between 5 and 7 years old, but this is only because so many patients are not identified until their first school medical examination. By this time histological changes have already occurred. If there is to be any improvement in the levels of risk for infertility or the development of germ cell tumours, earlier treatment is essential. Where the necessary expertise is available, treatment at one year of age would be ideal.

Medical treatment with gonadotrophin releasing hormone (GnRH) or human chorionic gonadotrophin (HCG) is advised by some enthusiasts but has not become generally accepted. GnRH 1.2 mg daily for 4 weeks or HCG 1500 units twice weekly for 3 weeks are said to make about 55 per cent of cryptorchids descend. Some of the reported cases may have had retractile testes. It seems a reasonable first line of treatment.

Surgical elongation of the cord to place the testis in the scrotum (orchiopexy) is the standard treatment. It may be complicated by damage to the blood supply or the vas, especially in very young patients, so it is not an operation that should be delegated to an inexperienced surgeon.

Torsion of the testis

The normal testis and epididymis are partly invested in tunica vaginalis. If the tunica is attached to the lower cord the testis and epididymis are effectively swinging free on the cord. When this abnormality is present the long axis of the testis lies horizontally in the scrotum when the patient is standing. It is known as the bell clapper deformity and is nearly always bilateral.

On its own it causes no problems. However, the testis may twist on its cord, stopping first the venous and then the arterial blood flow.

Torsion may be present at birth or occur shortly after. The infant presents with a red swollen scrotum. By the time the diagnosis is made the testis is nearly always dead and has to be removed.

However, torsion more commonly presents at 10-17 years of age. Thirty per cent of patients have a history of transient and self-limiting torsion before. Boys present with non-specific abdominal pain, vomiting and a red, swollen, tender scrotum. If the abdominal symptoms predominate, the diagnosis will be missed unless the genitalia are specifically examined.

Very urgent treatment is required. Operation within 5 hours of onset can save 80 per cent of testes, but by 10 hours less than 20 per cent can be saved. Torsion is by far the commonest cause of acute scrotal symptoms and signs in pubertal boys. In practice, no investigations help in the diagnosis and all suspected cases should be explored without delay.

At operation the cord is untwisted. If the testis is viable it is returned to the scrotum and sutured to the scrotal wall to prevent recurrence. Non-viable testes are removed. Because the bell clapper deformity is bilateral, the other side should always be fixed at the same operation.

Hydrocoele

The potential space between the tunica vaginalis and the testis may become filled with fluid at any age. The resulting scrotal swelling is, obviously, cystic. Because the testis is almost completely surrounded by the fluid it is impalpable. The swelling is easily transilluminated. The majority of hydrocoeles are idiopathic, but a small number are caused by testicular injury or inflammation.

The fluid can be aspirated with a small needle to give temporary relief. Curative treatment consists of surgical excision of the bulk of the tunica and oversewing of the free edge (Jaboulay's operation).

Epididymal cysts

The testis and the head of the epididymis join *in utero* by the union of 20 or more tubules which grow towards each other. Those that fail to meet may develop into cysts at any age but usually not before puberty.

Epididymal cysts are palpable separately from the testicle. If they fill with clear fluid (the common variety) they transilluminate. The minority contain spermatic debris which does not easily transilluminate.

They should not be aspirated as the fluid is highly irritative. They are easily removed surgically.

13

Male infertility and impotence

Infertility

Infertility probably affects up to 10 per cent of marriages, though not all couples are sufficiently troubled to seek medical help. For most couples, however, the gradual realization that they are unable to fulfil the role that society considers natural for them is extremely painful. The trauma is often compounded by the programme of investigation that is set in motion – prolonged and often unrewarding.

Physiology

The production, in the female, of ova and their passage through the genital tract are dealt with in *Reproduction and the Fetus* by A.L.R. Findlay. In the male, fertility depends on production of sperm in the testes and their passage through the vas to the seminal vesicles where other components are added to make semen (See Fig. 13.1). Male infertility is caused by failure of this system, though failure of delivery – impotence – can be another reason for failure to conceive.

Sperm are produced by the seminiferous tubules under the influence of follicle stimulating hormone (FSH) secreted by the pituitary gland. There is a negative feedback by inhibin produced by normally functioning tubules.

There is a very wide range of normal sperm production. Most laboratories accept 20 million sperm/ml as the lowest limit of normal, with at least 60 per cent of sperm showing progressive motility and less than 40 per cent being morphologically abnormal. However, there are many examples of fertile men with motile counts of 0.5 million/ml and infertile men with counts of 40 million/ml or more. Neither the count nor the ability of sperm to move forward indicate normal physiology: newer tests such as the ability of sperm to penetrate the zona-free hamster oocyte may prove a better guide in the future. At present the important distinction is between those who have sperm present and those who do not (azoospermia). Azoospermia may occur either because no sperm are made or because they cannot escape from the testes.

Azoospermia with normal FSH implies an obstructive aetiology, while high FSH implies non-functioning tubules. Low FSH is associated with endocrine disease, but is rare.

Infertility 137

Pituitary failure (rare): Low FSH and LH, low testosterone. Oligo- or azoospermia

FSH stimulates testosterone

Negative feedback with inhibin

Open bladder neck: Normal FSH, LH and testosterone. Normal testes. Retrograde ejaculation into bladder. Normal sperm in urine

Testicular failure: High FSH and LH. Testosterone usually normal. Small testes. Oligo- or azoospermia

Impotence or other sexual dysfunction may present as infertility

Obstruction in epididymis, vas or prostate: Normal FSH, LH and testosterone. Normal testes. Azoospermia.

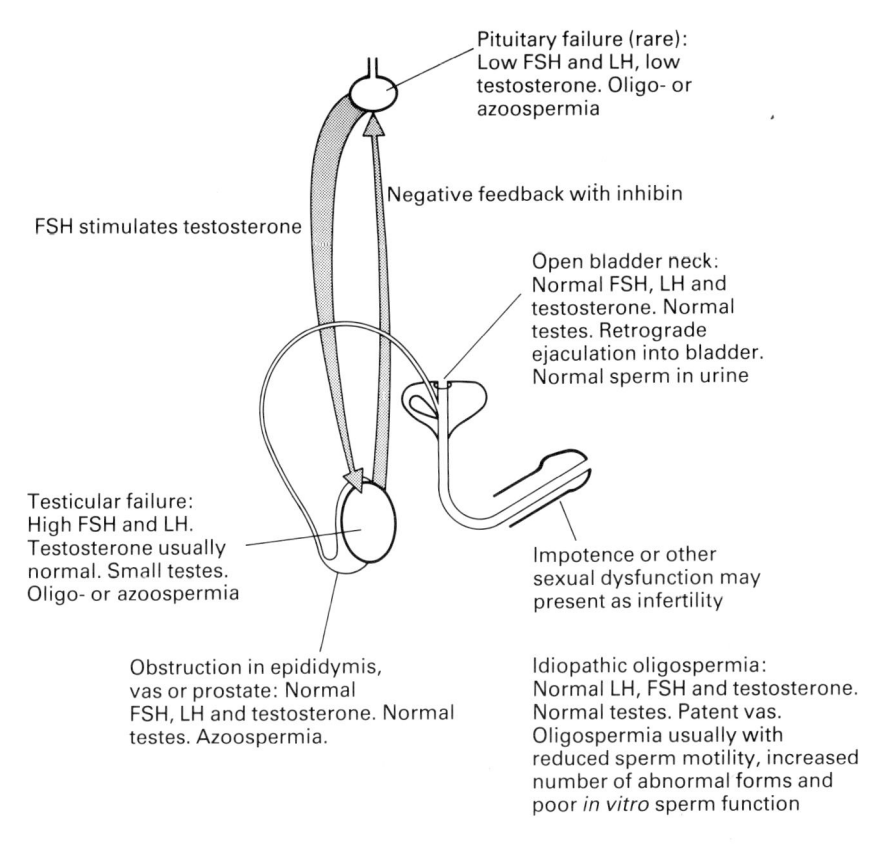

Idiopathic oligospermia: Normal LH, FSH and testosterone. Normal testes. Patent vas. Oligospermia usually with reduced sperm motility, increased number of abnormal forms and poor *in vitro* sperm function

Fig. 13.1 Findings in male infertility.

Obstructive azoospermia, that is occurring with normal FSH and normal sized testes, can be due to lesions anywhere between the epididymis and the ejaculatory ducts.

A low sperm count is associated with poorly functioning seminiferous tubules and normal or high FSH. Although some causes are known, most are idiopathic. Likewise, low motility has few treatable causes.

History

Infertility must always be regarded as a joint problem and both partners must be investigated initially. The first division of patients is into those who have had children (or pregnancies) before and those who have not: primary and secondary infertility. The circumstances of previous pregnancies give several clues to the cause of the presenting infertility: clearly if the husband has fathered children by an earlier marriage he is unlikely to require extensive investigation.

A sexual history is essential. It is probably not worth while to investigate couples who have been having unprotected intercourse for less than two years.

138 Male infertility and impotence

There is a close correlation between the length of involuntary infertility (the 'trying time') and the subsequent birth of a child: when the trying time has been 48 months and there is a mobile sperm count of 2 million/ml or more, over one-third of men will father a child in the ensuing year.

However, this rule of thumb must be balanced against the social changes of the last 20 years. With so many couples postponing their first attempts at pregnancy until their late twenties, infertility is becoming a problem later in a woman's reproductive life. Investigation may last a year or more and must not be allowed to carry the couple beyond the age at which pregnancy (or possibly adoption) is reasonable.

Occasionally it is found that couples do not know the fertility cycle and have not been having intercourse at the appropriate time. Other sexual difficulties or even impotence may be uncovered by a clinician who has the skill and time to ask the right questions.

A past history of groin or pelvic surgery, particularly for undescended testes, is relevant. Venereal disease or pelvic inflammatory disease may cause vasal or tubal obstruction, but it may not be possible to get this history when the partners are interviewed together.

Examination and investigation

Both partners must be examined. In clinics specializing in infertility, a gynaecologist and urologist usually work together. To indicate a positive attitude, such clinics are usually called 'Fertility Clinics'. The female aspects are dealt with in *Gynaecology, Obstetrics and the Neonate* by S.J. Steele.

The examination of the male partner should identify any major general problems that might be a bar to fertility, rare as they may be. There is an association between some forms of chronic bronchitis and infertility; it is thought to be due to a defect in the action of the cilia in bronchiolar and epididymal mucosa (Young's syndrome). Chromosomal anomalies usually produce a characteristic appearance: for example, Klinefelter's syndrome patients (44 XYY) have tall stature and very small soft testes. Penile abnormalities, unless very gross, do not cause infertility, and when they do it is usually due to problems of delivery of semen. Hypospadias and epispadias are not associated with infertility.

The scrotal contents must be examined in a warm room. The testes are normally 3–4 cm long, 2–3 cm in diameter and of firm consistency. The epididymis is easily felt attached in the long axis of the testis and continuing as the vas. Bilateral undescended testes persisting into adult life are incompatible with fertility.

Varicocele describes a collection of tortuous, dilated veins around the spermatic cord and tunica vaginalis. Ninety-five per cent occur on the left, 5 per cent are bilateral. The frequently-stated relationship between varicocele and infertility remains unproven. Varicocele is common and the incidence seems to be the same in fertile and infertile men. However, in infertile men with varicocele and no other recognizable cause for infertility, ligation of varicocele is followed by pregnancy sufficiently often to make the procedure worth while. It has been suggested that patients with free reflux from the testicular vein to the varicocele are most likely to benefit.

It is ideal for both partners to attend the same clinic for investigation. If this is not possible there must be close cooperation between the two clinics so that unnecessary investigations are avoided. For the man, the essential investigation is analysis of at least one, and preferably three, specimens of semen. The specimen must be produced by masturbation after three days of sexual abstinence and collected into a sterile, inert container. It must be kept at body temperature and examined within two hours of production. However, there is a wide range of 'normality' and the result is of little prognostic significance.

Sperm-agglutinating antibodies have been found in the serum and seminal plasma of both fertile and infertile men. They are also found after vasectomy, the titre rising with the passing years. Although the incidence and the titres are higher in infertile men, their significance is uncertain. Treatment with high-dose steroids is said to have produced some pregnancies, but final proof is lacking. Severe complications such as acute peptic ulceration and avascular hip necrosis can occur with this treatment.

Management

Azoospermia

Azoospermia from endocrine disease is covered by Steele in *Gynaecology, Obstetrics and the Neonate*. The only obstructive lesion worth correcting is the vasal obstruction close to the epididymis which usually follows gonorrhoea. It is identified by the presence on vasography of dilated epididymal tubules and a normal distal vas. It is treated by anastomosing some dilated epidymal tubules to the vas.

Low sperm count, or normal sperm count with infertility

Because there is a poor correlation between the sperm count and eventual paternity, it is difficult to give couples accurate advice. Low motility may be caused by chronic bacterial prostatitis as confirmed on culture of expressed prostatic secretion. Successful treatment with antibiotics may improve motility and allow pregnancy. Beyond this, there is no treatment of proven value to increase the sperm count or to make apparently non-functioning sperm produce a pregnancy. It has been said that testes should be 2 degrees (Celsius) cooler than normal body temperature: to this end a varicocele may be ligated, tight pants and very hot baths avoided.

Assuming that the female partner is normal, couples should be advised that conception is possible, but becomes less likely with each passing year. The alternative possibilities should be discussed. Artificial insemination by donor is available. Donors are matched for race and general family characteristics, but, except in a few centres in America, no other attempt is made to select especially desirable features. Adoption remains a possibility, but the number of babies available has fallen in recent years.

Once the treatments with a reasonable prospect of success have been tried in either partner, doctors and patients should strongly resist the temptation to carry on with increasingly forlorn experimental investigations and drugs.

140 Male infertility and impotence

Impotence

In common usage, the word 'impotence' means an inability to achieve an erection in response to appropriate sexual stimulation. However, such failure of the obvious manifestation of arousal is usually part of a more general failure of sexual function. It is a very common problem in the world at large and is poorly managed by most doctors. Normal sexual function depends on coordination between central and peripheral nervous systems, the vascular and the endocrine systems. Failure of any part will cause 'impotence'.

Mechanisms of normal erection

Neural factors

Erection may occur either through psychogenic stimulation or through a reflex pathway.

The psychogenic pathway begins in the cerebral cortex through erotic stimulation of specific centres: 'what turns you on'. The stimulus may be of any of the senses – visual, tactile, auditory, etc. – or may be imaginary. In humans specific erection and copulatory centres probably lie in the medial dorsal nucleus of the thalamus and in the medial septopreoptic region. The exact neural pathway is unknown, but is either through the sympathetic nerves from T12 to L3 or through the parasympathetic plexus from S2 to S4 (see Fig. 13.2).

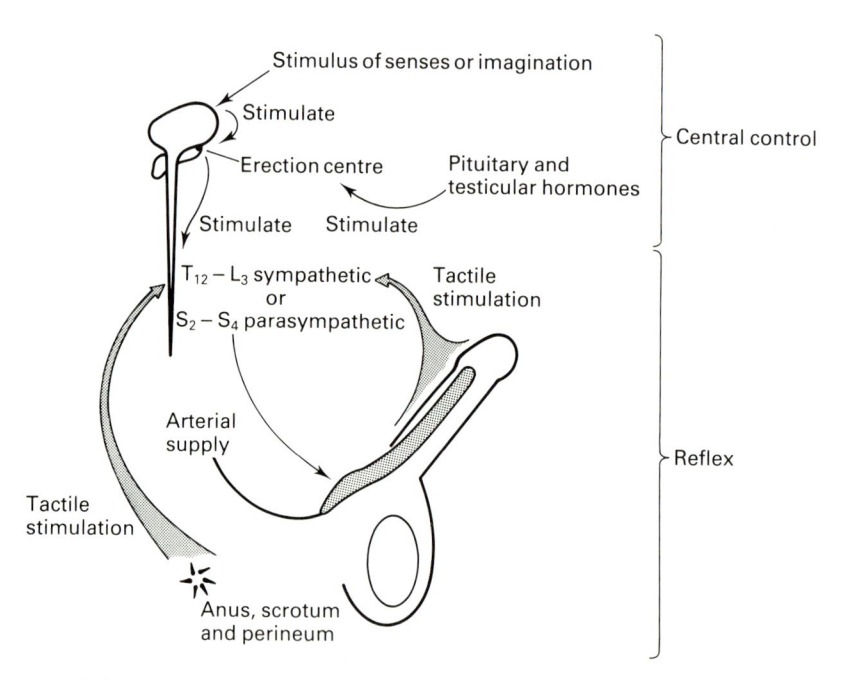

Fig. 13.2 Erectile pathways.

Peripheral erection centres can be found in the sympathetic thoracolumbar area and in the sacral parasympathetic area.

The reflex pathway is initiated by stimulation of receptors in the external genitalia, bladder or rectum. Afferent neurones travel in the pudendal nerves and the efferents in the sacral parasympathetic nerves.

Both pathways travel through the pelvic plexus of nerves lying between the rectum and prostate.

Initiating an erection, especially at the appropriate time, is not nearly as simple as this description implies. In paraplegics, reflex erections occur providing the neural pathway is intact. For all other men, the two systems interact and the overall cerebral stimulus may be inhibitory: conscious and subconscious stimuli may swamp the straightforward erotic stimuli so that the net effect is to prevent erection. Thus experiences and mores acquired in early life and stored in the subconscious may be a cause of impotence in adulthood.

Vascular factors

Erection occurs when the erectile tissue of the corpora cavernosa becomes engorged with blood. An artificial erection can be produced by perfusing the corpora with saline at over 20 ml/minute through an infusion needle. It is disputed whether natural erection occurs by increased arterial inflow, by decreased venous outflow, or by 'trapping' of blood in erectile tissue. There is experimental and pathological evidence to support all three theories, but no categorical proof.

Erectile tissue is mainly composed of vascular spaces, smooth muscle and bundles of elastic tissue. A current, favoured theory holds that relaxation of the smooth muscle bundles reduces the pressure in the vascular spaces, so that blood is drawn into the spaces. The engorgement may be maintained either by the elastic bundles keeping the spaces open or by 'baffles' in the venous endothelium which slow the outflow from the erectile tissue. 'Vascular' causes of impotence include inadequate blood supply and fibrosis of the erectile tissue sufficient to prevent expansion.

The neurotransmitter involved is probably neither cholinergic nor adrenergic. The most likely substance is vasoactive intestinal peptide (VIP). It is known to cause relaxation in vascular smooth muscle and is found in large concentrations in penile venous blood during erection. Large numbers of VIP nerve endings have been identified in corporeal vascular endothelium in potent men and reduced numbers in some impotent men. Intracorporeal injection of VIP produces erections.

Endocrine factors

Erection requires integrity of the hypothalamic–pituitary–gonadal axis. Endocrine failure may be implicated in as many as one-third of impotent men. (Details of the endocrinology appear in P. Daggett's book *Clinical Endocrinology*.) Many of the conditions causing impotence are congenital, such as Kallman's syndrome, hypogonadotrophic eunuchoidism, the Prader–Willi syndrome, and hypogonadism. Acquired lesions include hypogonadism from injury or infection, hyperprolactinaemia, panhypopituitarism and feminizing testicular tumours.

Impotence also occurs in some cases of endocrine disease not affecting the main hypothalamic-pituitary-gonadal axis. Thyrotoxicosis, hypothyroidism, Cushing's syndrome and Addison's disease are the commonest. Leydig cell function is altered, either directly or indirectly in these conditions, but the mechanisms are not well understood. Impotence does not occur in all cases. Chronic renal failure and alcoholic cirrhosis are commonly associated with impotence; the mechanisms are variable, and two or three distinct pathways have been identified in the two conditions.

Orgasm and ejaculation

Orgasm and ejaculation occur simultaneously but by different mechanisms.

Ejaculation describes the emission of seminal fluid. There is progressive, peristaltic contraction in the muscles from the epididymis, through the vasa to the prostatic ducts. Semen and prostatic fluid are deposited in the bulbar urethra and forcefully expelled by rhythmic contraction of the bulbospongiosus and perineal muscles. Reflex contraction of the bladder neck prevents retrograde flow into the bladder.

Orgasm is the subjective feeling of the ejaculation, the non-genital and emotional features of the end of intercourse. The intensity of orgasm is partly related to the volume of the ejaculate and its passage through the urethra. Patients who do not ejaculate owing to nerve damage, and those with retrograde ejaculation following prostatectomy, experience an orgasm of diminished intensity.

The neural centres and pathways of orgasm and ejaculation are less clearly defined than those for erection. The afferent stimulus is certainly very variable and includes direct sensory nerves in the genitalia and stimulation of the higher senses, such as hearing, smell and sight. The stimulatory effect of imagination and the inhibitory effects of conscious and subconscious thoughts are also important. The main efferent pathway is through thoracolumbar sympathetic nerves. Bilateral (but not unilateral) sympathectomy abolishes ejaculation: an important consideration in planning the management of the retroperitoneal nodes in young men with testicular neoplasia.

Orgasm is usually followed by detumescence and a period during which there is no response to sexual stimuli. Failure of detumescence after any erection is rare and leads to the important condition of priapism.

'Organic' versus 'psychogenic' impotence

The complex physiology of sexual function makes it difficult to distinguish between psychological and neurovascular causes of impotence. Even in a case with absolutely clear-cut aetiology, the interaction between the two mechanisms is such that a 'cure' remains elusive. For example, the insertion of a penile prosthesis in a young man with nerve damage following pelvic fracture does not always restore emotionally satisfactory sexual function.

When erections occur spontaneously – such as during sleep or in the early morning with a full bladder – but not at the time of intercourse, it might be thought that the cause is psychogenic. Recent research has shown that most cases are multifactorial. Although identification of principal causes helps in management, a strict division of all cases into 'organic' and 'psychogenic' groups is neither possible nor desirable. The finding that the number of VIP nerve endings is reduced in the corpora of men with organic and supposedly 'psychogenic' impotence underlines this point.

Patient history

Most doctors manage impotence badly. Although it is true that most cases of impotence lack specific treatments, much of the blame for bad management lies with the doctor. In the past, medical training included little about sex and information was gleaned from conversations in the hospital bar: doctors were thus little better educated than their patients. Added to this ignorance has been the inability of doctors to discuss sex openly and in terms that ordinary patients can understand. All this is very surprising considering that the enormous role of sexuality in life has been recognized for over 100 years.

To have any success in treating impotence the clinician must be able to draw a good history from a patient who is usually discussing a subject on which he has never spoken before except in a 'barrack-room' context. Time and patience are of the essence. In a few cases the history will reveal an obvious cause that is recognized as 'organic': a history of pelvic surgery likely to have damaged the prostatic neural plexus, for example. Impotence is almost invariable after cystoprostatectomy for bladder carcinoma, and follows pelvic fracture with rupture of the membranous urethra in 50–65 per cent of cases. Some drugs, including stilboestrol, cimetidine and hypnotics, are causes of, or associated with, impotence (see Fig. 13.3).

Peripheral neuropathy (as in diabetes) and peripheral vascular disease both cause impotence, though the precise mechanism is not known. In Leriche's syndrome patients complain of intermittent claudication and impotence. Alcoholism is an important cause of impotence even before it has caused other problems.

Most cases, however, lack such distinctive histories. For these, step-by-step progression is often necessary to discover which aspects of sexual function are abnormal. If there is failure of erection it is essential to discover if erections *ever* occur (for example, in the morning on waking; if they occur in anticipation of intercourse but disappear on penetration of the vagina; or whether intercourse is possible but with less frequency than desired). It must be remembered that there are many causes for dissatisfaction with the sexual act other than erectile impotence.

Examination

Like the history, the examination seldom reveals an obvious cause for impotence. Relevant findings include general signs of endocrine disease, including abnormalities of secondary sexual characteristics; liver disease; abdominal scars; painful lesions of the penis or scrotum, especially balanitis and

144 Male infertility and impotence

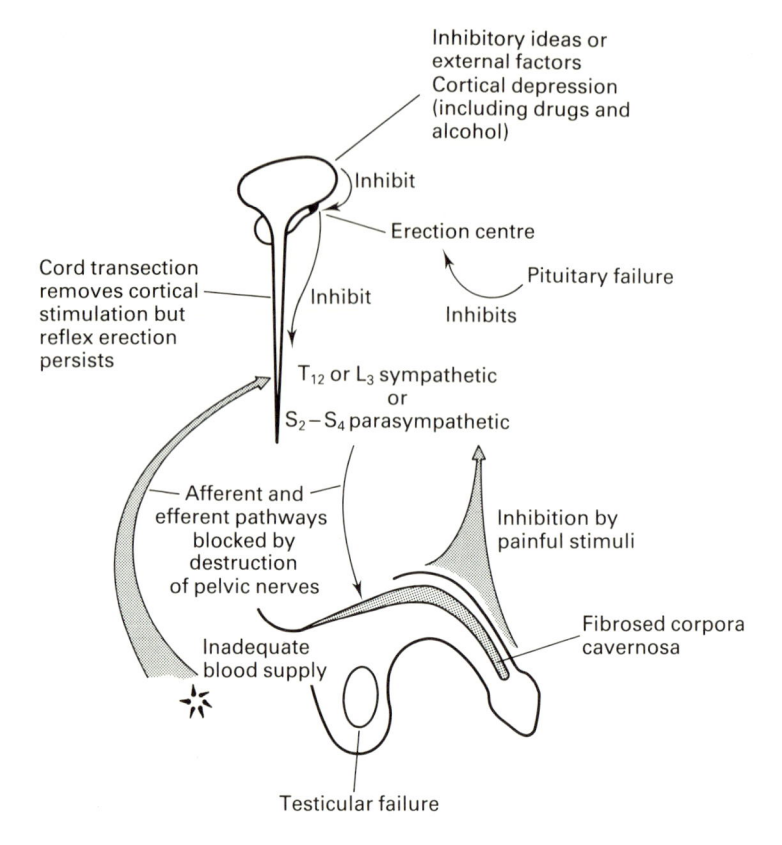

Fig. 13.3 The causes of impotence.

recurrently torn frenulum; signs of penile disease; poor condition of the vascular tree, especially in the lower limbs; and neurological abnormalities such as saddle anaesthesia and loss of lower limb vibration sense. On rectal examination, lack of tone in the anal sphincter may be the first clue to neurological disease. Extensive pelvic cancer, especially prostatic, may be a cause of impotence.

Anatomical anomalies of the penis are not, in themselves, causes of impotence; anxiety about such anomalies may be. As an extreme example, young men born with the exstrophy/epispadias complex of anomalies have a short, stumpy penis that seldom exceeds 5 cm in erect length: they have high libido and function sexually to their own and their established partner's satisfaction, though they have fewer partners overall than age-matched controls. The 'normal' penis, like all other organs of the body, is of variable size, and even at the bottom of the normal range has normal physiological function. Some men focus their feelings of sexual inadequacy on their allegedly abnormal penis: occasionally, very severely disturbed men attempt to amputate the object of their dissatisfaction. Men who believe that their penis is too small need much reassurance and support.

Investigation

The large number of causes makes the investigation of impotence difficult. Ideally, patients should be managed in a clinic jointly by urologists and psychiatrists. The prevalence of the complaint would certainly justify this organization, but for the present resources do not permit it.

Preliminary screening by history and examination should identify three main groups:

(1) those with irreversible erectile impotence, usually due to destruction of pelvic nerves, though sometimes due to vascular disease or extensive penile fibrosis following priapism;
(2) men with signs or symptoms suggestive of specific disease, usually endocrine, with impotence associated (previously unrecognized alcoholism is probably the commonest condition in this group);
(3) all the rest: a large group.

In practice it would be easy to be swamped by the final group. It is useful to subdivide it, in a simple way, into those whose sexual function is comparable to that of a peer group but whose perception of their performance leads to a complaint of impotence; and those who are distinctly different from their peers. This is an artificial distinction, but it does save many men from undergoing a barrage of investigations with almost no prospect of 'curative' treatment at the end.

The chief difficulty of the foregoing division is in defining the 'normal' for any particular peer group. At the simplest level, some men have unrealistic expectations based on their reading of modern novels and sexy magazines, watching films and discussions in the pub. Scientifically, we have to rely on the widely quoted work of Masters and Johnson and of Kinsey who surveyed essentially normal populations, and of sexual rehabilitation units that deal with essentially abnormal patients. People have intercourse much less often than popular myth suggests, as the figures in Table 13.1 show. The incidence of impotence in otherwise normal men rises from 1.5 per cent at 40 to 25 per cent at 70 years old, and is correlated with falling testosterone levels (though remaining in the normal range) and rising gonadotrophin levels suggesting gradual Leydig cell failure. An American survey of patients presenting with urological cancer suggested that normal married couples have some regular sexual activity that they consider important until the man is 70. Thereafter activity and interest fall off rapidly, usually with the man leading the way.

Table 13.1 One analysis of the percentage of men having intercourse more than once a week (Data from Pearlman, C.K. and Kobashi, L.I. (1972). Frequency of intercourse in men, *J. Urol.*, **107**, 298–301)

Age	20	20–49	50–59	60–69	70–79	80+
%	88	80	68	50	25	10

146 Male infertility and impotence

For some men, therefore, sympathetic explanation of the realities of life may be all that is required.

Endocrine investigations

Patients with signs or symptoms of endocrine disease require specific investigation. For those with no ready diagnosis (from group 3 above), a preliminary screening of blood investigations should include haemoglobin, electrolytes, urea and creatinine, liver function tests, blood sugar, testosterone and prolactin.

Vascular investigations

A high arterial blood flow is necessary to initiate an erection and this may not be achieved in arteriopaths. The simplest guide is to measure the penile blood pressure (using a small cuff and Doppler stethoscope) and compare it with the arm blood pressure: the penile systolic blood pressure should be the same as or greater than the mean systemic arterial pressure (one-third of the pulse pressure plus the diastolic pressure).

Neurological investigations

There are no specific neurological tests for impotence. The progressive loss of erectile capacity caused by autonomic neuropathy may be associated with bladder dysfunction. A cystometrogram may define the lesion more clearly. Diabetes is the commonest cause.

Corporeal biopsy to look for alterations in nerve endings microscopically is experimental at present, but may become routine when its place has been defined.

In some cases it may be useful to determine whether spontaneous erections occur during sleep, especially during rapid-eye-movement sleep. If any erections occur, the implication is that neural and vascular supplies are intact. Nocturnal tumescence can most simply be identified by the postage stamp test. A strip of stamps is stuck around the circumference of the penis: if erection occurs the perforations will be broken in the morning. A more scientific version of this test has a stretch-sensitive loop around the penis connected to a recorder: the frequency and extent of erections are thus known.

Radiological investigations

Penile curvature (chordee) may cause sexual dysfunction. Patients are not normally impotent because penile tumescence occurs, but the chordee prevents penetration. This may be even more distressing than true impotence. Peyronie's disease is the commonest cause: in this condition benign fibrous plaques develop in the tunica albuginea and slowly shrink, causing progressive curvature. It is often helpful to ask patients to produce a photograph of their erection.

Where there is doubt about the type of curvature, especially if it follows

Impotence 147

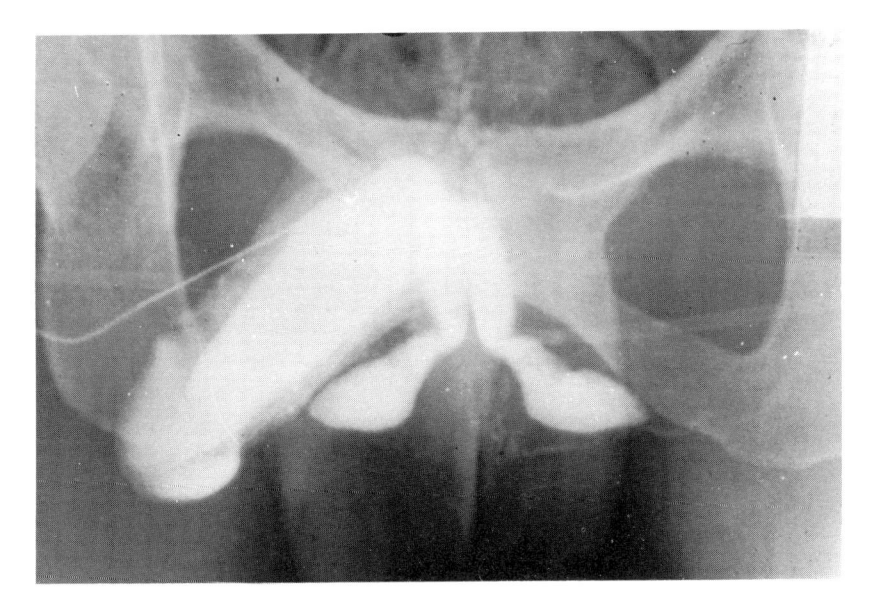

Fig. 13.4 Cavernosogram of a normal penis.

trauma, surgery or priapism, cavernosography is indicated. Radiographs are taken after infusing dilute vascular contrast medium directly into the corpora cavernosa (Fig. 13.4). The anatomy of the penile blood supply can be investigated by means of a transcutaneous selective pudendal arteriogram. It is indicated only in carefully selected patients and as part of the investigation of their general arterial disease.

Treatment

Prosthesis

Prostheses can be inserted in the corpora. There are two main types: inflatable and rigid. Rigid prostheses are silicone rods, which leave the patient with a permanent erection. One variety, designed by Jonas, is less rigid and has a core of silver which allows the penis to be bent downwards when not being used for intercourse. Prostheses of this type are simple and relatively cheap. Providing the right size is used and they do not become infected, the level of complications is acceptable (Fig. 13.5).

An inflatable prosthesis has been designed by Brantley-Scott and is widely used. It consists of two silicone cylinders which are put in the corpora and are inflated from a subcutaneous reservoir by a small finger-operated pressure pump sited in the scrotum. The device is expensive and liable to infection and to mechanical failure. However, many surgeons consider it the treatment of choice in 'organic impotence', especially following pelvic surgery or fractures.

The place of prosthetic surgery in the management of impotence that is not

148 *Male infertility and impotence*

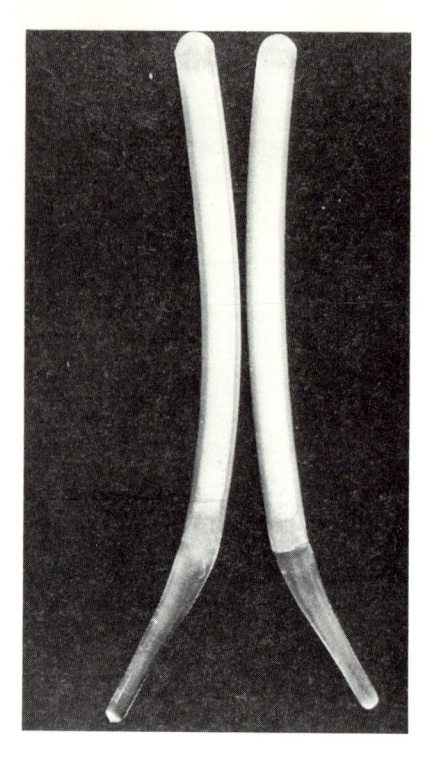

Fig. 13.5 Implantable penile prosthesis for impotence.

clearly 'organic' remains controversial. Many cases of impotence are multifactorial, and quite marked psychiatric symptoms may be secondary to fairly minor organic causes of impotence. When impotence is but the presenting symptom of extensive psychosexual or marital problems, insertion of a prosthesis is unlikely to be helpful. All patients being considered for prosthetic surgery require careful counselling which should, if possible, involve the partner.

Other surgery

When a specific penile anomaly responsible for impotence is found, corrective surgery may be possible. Penile curvature is the commonest cause. With a normal sized penis, shortening of the convex side of the curve is simplest. An appropriately sized ellipse of tunica albuginea is excised and the defect closed (Nesbitt's procedure). If the penis is abnormally short already, as in epispadias, it is desirable to lengthen the concave aspect of the curvature. This may be done by incising each tunica around two-thirds of its circumference, straightening the curvature and inserting an appropriately sized ellipse of tissue such as tunica vaginalis or lyophilized cadaveric dura mater.

Painful penile lesions such as phimosis with recurrent balanitis and recurrently torn frenulum may cause erectile failure. Corrective surgery is usually curative.

Vascular surgery to correct impotence is difficult and rarely indicated. Surgery for lesions in the abdominal aorta and common iliacs for intermittent claudication may improve erectile function, but not always. Vascular surgery distal to the origin of the internal iliac artery may worsen impotence by further diverting blood flow into the legs. In no case should vascular surgery be undertaken to improve blood flow without first considering the rest of the arterial tree.

The only neurological disease likely to be treated surgically is spinal cord compression, especially by prolapsed intervertebral disc. Impotence from this cause is usually associated with urinary retention and is rare.

Drug therapy

If a specific endocrinopathy is identified, replacement therapy usually restores potency. Direct, self-injection of the corpora cavernosa with papaverine produces an erection for two hours and is a very useful form of management when no other is available. Testosterone therapy, even in the elderly with lower blood levels of testosterone, is useless.

Primary psychiatric disease, especially depression, may be associated with impotence. Successful treatment, including drug treatment, may help. However, most of the commonly used drugs, including tricyclics, monoamine oxidase inhibitors, benzodiazepines and phenothiazines, have impotence as a recognized side-effect.

Psychosexual therapy

During the investigation of impotence the clinician must form an impression of the relative importance of 'organic' and 'psychogenic' factors in each case. If impotence is found to be a symptom of a severe psychiatric illness, psychiatric referral is indicated.

For the majority of patients, especially those with an established partner, impotence can be traced to relatively minor anxieties about one or more aspects of sexuality. Perhaps the greatest problem in managing these problems is to get both partners to accept that there is a problem that can be treated. The techniques used to identify and treat such problems are beyond the scope of this book. In recent years, the prognosis for this type of impotence has improved considerably.

Priapism

Priapism describes a painful, non-physiological erection which does not detumesce spontaneously. Untreated it eventually resolves over several weeks with fibrous replacement of the corpora which causes impotence.

Most cases follow the chain of events shown in Fig. 13.6. Initiating events, which can occur at several points in the cycle, include spinal cord transection, sickle cell disease, leukaemia, multiple myeloma, malignant hypertension and

150 Male infertility and impotence

Mechanism of priapism (after Hinman)

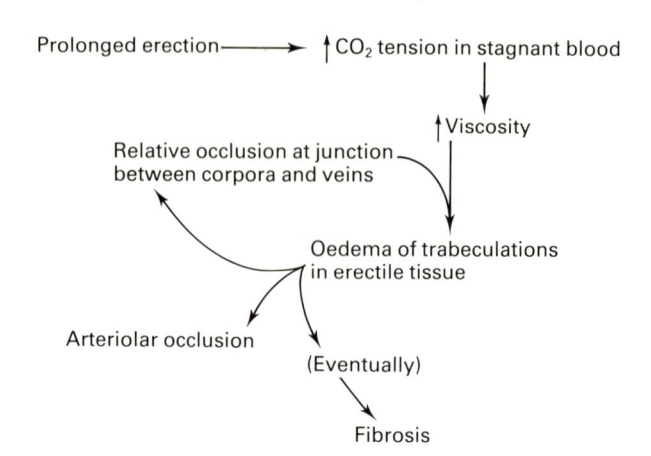

Prolonged erection ⟶ ↑CO_2 tension in stagnant blood
↓
↑Viscosity
Relative occlusion at junction between corpora and veins
↓
Oedema of trabeculations in erectile tissue
↓
Arteriolar occlusion
↓
(Eventually)
↓
Fibrosis

Fig. 13.6 Mechanism of priapism.

prostatitis. In the United Kingdom most cases are idiopathic and follow prolonged sexual stimulation.

Urgent surgical treatment is required. The corpora are thoroughly irrigated to remove the stagnant blood. Thereafter a corporovenous fistula is constructed, usually with the saphenous vein, to ensure drainage.

About 50 per cent of patients are successfully detumesced in the long term, but fewer if treatment is delayed for more than 24 hours. Only about a half of these retain normal potency.

14

Tubular disorders

The tubular mechanisms involved in the modification of the glomerular filtrate have been described (Hladky and Rink, Chapters 6, 7 and 8). The left ventricle provides the energy for filtration and the tubular cells themselves generate the energy for the modification of the filtrate.

In clinical nephrology the emphasis is on glomerular filtration – its measurement and the consequences that follow its reduction. This bias stems from a difficulty in accurately measuring intricate tubular mechanisms in patients. In Chapter 1 details of some tubular function tests relating to concentration and acidification are described, but it requires constant intravenous infusion techniques to produce an arterial steady state, with careful urine collections via a bladder catheter, to assess active transport mechanisms and provide tubular maxima (T_m) values. These are mainly research procedures and play little part in routine practice. Despite these limitations valuable, if incomplete, information can be obtained, allowing tubular defects to be recognized and treated.

There are two main categories:

(1) specific, inherited, defects of tubular transport;
(2) tubular problems that are secondary to general pathology – acquired defects.

In this chapter the common defects in group 1 will be described and an outline of those in group 2 given, as the specific defects are covered when the subject is described in greater detail elsewhere in the text.

Specific tubular defects

Hypophosphataemic rickets

Filtered phosphate is mainly reabsorbed by the distal tubule and is under the control of the parathyroid hormone (PTH). There is no evidence of tubular secretion. In hypophosphataemic rickets the T_m for phosphate is low and the urinary loss is therefore high, a state of affairs which is not influenced by PTH.

This defect is congenital and linked to the X-chromosome with a varying degree of penetrance. The children have a low plasma phosphate and a normal calcium, growth is stunted and the legs are bowed. It is difficult to account for

152 Tubular disorders

the osteomalacia and ligament calcification that occur by what is known of the tubular defects.

Treatment is not very effective, but some patients respond to regular phosphate replacement and the judicious use of vitamin D, though care must be taken to avoid hypercalcaemia.

Pseudohypoparathyroidism

In a small group of patients tubules are refractory to the influence of PTH. Phosphate reabsorption is excessive, producing elevated plasma levels and a secondary reduction in calcium. The patients are short of stature, intellectually impaired and have ectopic calcification in brain and soft tissue.

Management centres on maintaining a normal serum calcium by means of oral vitamin D.

Vitamin D dependent rickets

The sequelae which follow the lack of active vitamin D production by the kidney are described in Chapter 4, covering renal osteodystrophy in relation to chronic renal failure. A similar sequence of events occurs in the first few months of life owing to the lack of a tubular enzyme, 1-α-hydroxylase. The genetic defect is autosomal recessive, and its early detection is important as treatment with the active form of vitamin D, ^{125}dihydroxycholicalciferol (1α vitamin D), has greatly improved the prognosis in these patients.

Cystinuria

Amino acids are freely filtered and reabsorbed by active transport, and abnormal urinary losses can be detected by paper chromatography. Improved analytical techniques allow identification and accurate measurement of individual amino acids to be made.

In health the essential amino acids are almost completely reabsorbed, but some of the non-essential amino acids – such as glycine, taurine and histidine – can be detected in normal urine. Patients with cystinuria cannot reabsorb cystine, ornithine, lysine and arginine, but it is only the first that presents clinical problems; the increased urinary excretion of cystine leads to stone formation because this amino acid is relatively insoluble. The stones are faintly radio-opaque and, as in all cases of stone disease, can produce obstruction, infection and impaired renal function.

The treatment of this autosomal recessive disorder depends on maintaining a 24-hour production of a dilute urine to prevent crystal deposition and stone growth. Cystine is more soluble in an alkaline medium, and so oral sodium bicarbonate may help. If these measures fail then penicillamine which forms a soluble complex with cystine, can be given. This drug must be used with care as it can produce glomerular damage, leading to proteinuria and a reduction in filtration.

It was hoped that extracorporeal lithotripsy would help these patients, but unfortunately these stones are refractory to this form of disintegration.

Specific tubular defects 153

Cystinosis

This rare, autosomal recessive condition should not be confused with cystinuria. In cystinosis, cystine causes damage by accumulating within cells, of which the renal tubular cell is an example. Tubular function is altered and there is inability to concentrate urine, a leakage of bicarbonate, phosphate and potassium, and failure to excrete hydrogen ions. Also, active vitamin D is not produced. Cystine accumulates in the cornea and other tissues, with the result that within a year the child does not thrive, and in extreme cases becomes dehydrated and acidotic.

Treatment in the long term is ineffective. However, careful fluid control, with oral sodium and potassium bicarbonate, partly correct the acidosis and potassium loss. These measures may prolong life, making renal transplantation a possibility.

Fanconi syndrome

In the late 1930s Fanconi described a series of patients with multiple tubular defects. Glycosuria, phosphaturia and aminoaciduria predominated. With time it became clear that some of these defects were secondary to heavy-metal poisoning, drug toxicity, etc.; but there are patients with no such history, and they represent the idiopathic familial form.

Again, replacement therapy and oral vitamin D to prevent osteomalacia are the basis of treatment.

Renal tubular acidosis

Tubular faults associated with the inability to produce an acid urine are usually acquired, but a rare congenital form does exist. Many groups of patients have been described, but the student need only consider two main types, distal tubular acidosis and proximal tubular acidosis.

Distal tubular acidosis

In this group the urine in the distal tubule cannot be acidified, either because free hydrogen ions are not secreted or because of immediate back diffusion. If urine of pH below 6.0 is never produced, then an acidification test will confirm the diagnosis.

Familial forms present as failure to thrive, but there is rapid clinical improvement when bicarbonate supplements are given.

Fine calcification throughout the renal parenchyma (nephrocalcinosis) occurs, and no explanation has been found for this deposition (Fig. 14.1). Other forms of nephrocalcinosis (shown in Table 14.1) are often associated with a failure to acidify.

Proximal tubular acidosis

This refers to the inability of the proximal tubule to reabsorb the filtered

154 Tubular disorders

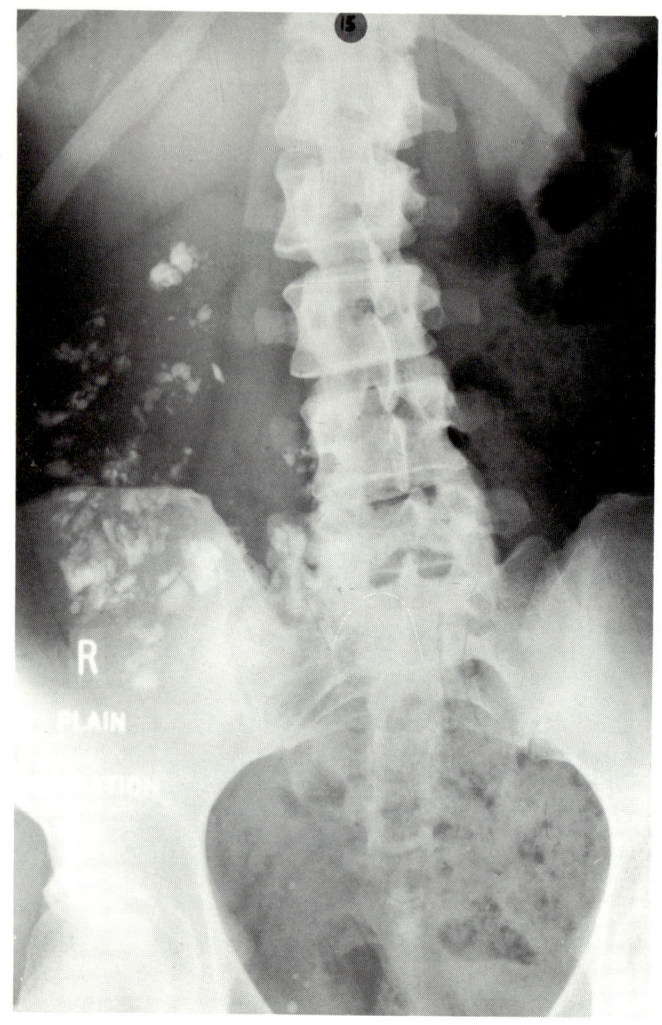

Fig. 14.1 A plain abdominal X-ray showing extensive nephrocalcinosis in a solitary right kidney.

Table 14.1 Common causes of nephrocalcinosis

Hyperparathyroidism	Papillary necrosis
Renal tubular acidosis	Oxalosis
Medullary sponge kidney	Sarcoidosis
Idiopathic hypercalciuria	Causes unknown
Milk alkali syndrome	

bicarbonate, and that generated in the tubular cells in the process of hydrogen ion generation. This abnormally low T_m for bicarbonate reabsorption means that the bulk of the filtered bicarbonate passes on to the distal tubule, where the production of hydrogen ions is insufficient to overcome the alkaline load and produce an acid urine.

This familial form, which presents in childhood as failure to thrive, is also associated with abnormal urinary losses of potassium and amino acid.

Along with substantial amounts of bicarbonate, potassium supplementation is also required. Acquired bicarbonate wasting may be found in cases of amyloidosis, analgesic damage and in the transplanted kidney.

Renal diabetes insipidus

In this familial, sex-linked condition the tubules do not respond to the antidiuretic hormone. Concentration is therefore not possible, leading if uncorrected to severe dehydration and hypotension. If a formal concentration test fails to produce a urine to high osmolality, then the response to injected desamino-D-8-arginine vasopressin (DDAVP) confirms that it is the tubules themselves that are at fault and not a defect in ADH production. DDAVP is a powerful synthetic derivative of vasopressin possessing antidiuretic activity, but it does not affect the cardiovascular system (i.e. it is not a vasopressor).

Treatment is aimed at preventing dehydration by ensuring an adequate fluid intake – a factor of critical importance in the newborn. In adult life the apparently paradoxical use of thiazide diuretics is often beneficial. It is thought that the chronic use of diuretics lowers the extracellular fluid volume, thus increasing the obligatory reabsorption of sodium and water in the proximal tubule, thereby reducing the volume delivered to the distal nephron, and thus reducing the urine volume.

Acquired tubular defects

Congenital tubular defects provide insight into normal tubular physiology and are of great importance to the paediatric nephrologist. More common, however, are the acquired defects encountered in adult patients. Acquired defects covered elsewhere in this book will only be mentioned briefly in this chapter.

The major components of the glomerular filtrate will be considered in turn: for normal mechanisms, see Hladky and Rink, Chapters 6 and 7.

Sodium

In chronic renal failure the glomerular tubular balance is maintained until the glomerular filtration rate has fallen to below 15 ml/minute. However, in some cases excessive sodium is lost (sodium-losing nephritis) and must be replaced. Inappropriate amounts are also lost following the relief of urinary tract obstruction and during the recovery, polyuric phase of acute renal failure.

The sodium retention which occurs in the nephrotic syndrome and in

156 Tubular disorders

cardiac failure is a normal response and the nephrons are behaving entirely appropriately.

Water

The major clinical feature is the inability to conserve water during times of dehydration and increased plasma osmolality. Assuming antidiuretic hormone is produced by the intact hypothalamic-pituitary pathway, it is the tubule that cannot respond. The following are the common factors producing this problem.

Chronic renal failure

This occurs when the increased filtered osmotic load overrides the normal concentrating mechanisms.

Obstruction

During recovery from complete or partial obstruction the tubules are refractory to antidiuretic hormone, and there is evidence of redistribution of intrarenal blood flow. The increased medullary blood flow may prevent the maintenance of the high interstitial osmolality that is essential for urine concentration.

Hypercalcaemia

Often associated with nephrocalcinosis, this may damage tubular cells, again rendering them refactory to the influence of antidiuretic hormone.

Hypokalaemia

Vacuolation of the tubular cells occurs with an effect similar to a raised calcium level.

Papillary necrosis

The medullary pyramids can be destroyed in patients who have consumed large amounts of analgesics (mainly phenacetin); this is analgesic nephropathy. Destruction of the hypertonic pyramids will clearly limit urine concentration. Similar damage can be produced by diabetes mellitus, malignant hypertension and sickle cell disease.

Potassium

Excessive loss will occur during the recovery phase of acute renal failure. Excessive losses may occur in primary or secondary hyperaldosteronism associated with congestive cardiac failure, the nephrotic syndrome and liver disease. Iatrogenic loss will occur during prolonged diuretic therapy.

Calcium

Seventy per cent of the filtered calcium is reabsorbed by the proximal tubule, the remainder being reabsorbed by the loop of Henle and the distal tubule. Hypercalciuria is thought to be a reflection solely of an increased calcium excretion, but it is clear that a tubular fault does exist whereby calcium is not reabsorbed, leading to excessive loss. This may be a factor in the production of renal calculi.

Magnesium

Well over 90 per cent of the filtered magnesium is reabsorbed, with the major site being the thick ascending loop of Henle. There is no tubular secretion.

Clinically, a low magnesium is often associated with excessive loss from the gastrointestinal tract during episodes of diarrhoea. Increased urinary loss does occur, again during the diuretic phase of acute renal failure following the relief of obstruction.

Several reports of excessive magnesium loss have been reported following renal transplantation, and certain drugs such as amphotericin and diuretics also produce inappropriate urinary losses.

Aminoaciduria

Amino acids may appear in the urine purely as a result of high plasma levels and an increased filtered load (e.g. phenylketonuria and advanced hepatic necrosis). The normal tubular reabsorption cannot cope with the increased load, and the amino acids appear in the urine. Tubular damage produced by heavy metals such as lead and mercury produce a general amino acid leak. In this case the tubular reabsorptive mechanism is impaired. Similar urinary losses occur with amyloid and myeloma. These urinary losses indicate tubular damage but are of little clinical significance.

Hydrogen ions

Acquired proximal tubular wasting of bicarbonate (type II) is a common occurrence in patients with amyloid, and occasionally follows transplantation and acetazolamide therapy, while a distal fault can occur with autoimmune disease such as SLE, Sjögren's syndrome and chronic active hepatitis. These conditions may also be associated with nephrocalcinosis.

Analgesic nephropathy and the use of such drugs as amphotericin are all associated with a similar lesion, and the tubular fault by and large is corrected when the drug is withdrawn.

15

Renal disease in general medicine

Diabetes mellitus

This condition which is a very common cause of chronic renal failure, presents particular management problems. The involvement of the small vessels produces widespread organ damage, and this microangiopathy occludes the arterioles and glomerular capillaries.

Descriptions of various histological features have been produced, but they probably just represent different stages of the same relentless destruction that will occur as long as the blood sugar remains high.

Traditionally, the classic form described by Kimmelsteil and Wilson is a thickening of the basement membrane and capillary walls with an eosinophilic material which aggregates into nodules in certain areas of the hypercellular glomerular tuft. Capillary damage allows fibrin leakage which may also appear as drops of eosinophilic material adherent to the capsule. These are given the obvious descriptive term of 'capsular drops'. Hyaline degeneration and occlusion of glomerular vessels leads to permanent glomerular sclerosis.

The functional changes resulting from this damage start with a leakage of protein into the filtrate. At first this is minimal and selective, but it can progress until a non-selective loss of 5-10 g/24 hours is achieved.

In the early stages the kidneys are large, with an increase in blood flow and glomerular filtration rate. As vascular damage occurs there is a progressive fall in the glomerular filtration rate. No clear explanation has emerged for this initial hyperfiltration.

Certain additional factors may coexist to speed functional decline:

(1) One or both renal arteries may be partially occluded with atheroma, producing poor perfusion.
(2) Uncontrolled hypertension may add to the vascular damage.
(3) Peripheral neuropathy may produce incomplete bladder emptying, and the residual urine may become infected.
(4) Papillary necrosis may lead to the shedding of a papilla, which can cause an obstruction. Papillary necrosis is thought to be produced by diabetic-induced vascular damage and appears to be associated with prolonged episodes of dehydration which may occur during hyperosmolar coma.
(5) Dehydration prior to an intravenous urogram, plus the toxic effect of

contrast media, may produce acute upon chronic failure. It is therefore important that contrast should be used with care and patients should not be subject to dehydration before investigation.
(6) An increase in platelet stickiness may produce a hypercoagulable state, thus adding to the vascular damage and occlusion.
(7) Associated coronary artery disease may produce poor left ventricular function. The resultant low cardiac output will lead to a reduction in glomerular filtration.
(8) Some patients of a particular HLA type can progress more rapidly into renal failure, suggesting that there is a genetic pre-disposition.

Prevention of the relentless renal damage is a major clinical problem. Careful blood sugar control throughout the 24-hour period is clearly very important, and future research may show that this will retard, if not prevent, the decline in function. The use of the new generation of insulins which contain no foreign protein may prevent immunological damage, and constant subcutaneous infusion achieved by small micropumps may be the treatment of the future.

Hypertensive control is the second most important factor. Here, beta-adrenergic blocking drugs plus modern vasodilators are useful. When beta-adrenergic blockade was first used some clinicians were concerned that if hypoglycaemia occurred the symptoms would be masked, and the return of blood sugar to normal would be delayed as the rate of gluconeogenesis is reduced. Experience has shown that these were mainly theoretical objections, and certainly the cardioselective drugs such as atenolol can be used safely.

Research continues into the value of reducing intravascular coagulation with antiplatelet drugs such as aspirin and dipyridamole. This is an important area of research. It is hoped that it will prove of clinical benefit, especially to juvenile diabetics who seem to pursue a relentless course to renal failure.

When end-stage renal failure is reached the problem of replacement therapy is also difficult. The patient may have other vascular complications such as coronary artery disease, intermittent claudication and retinal involvement which may have progressed to blindness; these are all factors that may make substitution therapy inappropriate. Vascular access for haemodialysis is often difficult, and recently the use of chronic ambulatory dialysis (CAPD) with intra-peritoneal insulin has been the treatment of choice.

Transplantation may also be difficult because of major vessel disease, and it is not surprising that the long-term graft survival is poor.

Obviously prevention is better than cure. While some units struggle with dialysis and transplantation, many are attempting to achieve good blood sugar control and correct haematological factors, hoping that progressive damage may be prevented.

Vasculitis

There are a number of diseases which in the past have been described as separate entities but which, it is now clear, share a common pathology, namely immunologically induced vascular damage. The size of vessel and organ involved varies, giving rise to a series of clinical entities which may fit the original historical description, but often there is a great deal of overlap so that the patient's clinical description will not fit exactly. The common clinical entities are systemic lupus erythematosus (SLE), polyarteritis nodosa, Wegener's granulomatosis, Henoch-Schönlein purpura, systemic sclerosis and rheumatoid arthritis. The kidneys may escape, but if they arc involved the long-term prognosis is generally poor.

It is thought that the vascular damage is produced by the deposition of immune complexes. The trigger to producing antibody is uncertain, but bacterial and viral infection may be responsible. Drugs may not only provide a similar antigen but may so alter tissue protein that it becomes antigenic. In the case of SLE the antibody is directed against nucleic acid.

With the common background of immunological damage several clinical features are common. Examination of the skin may reveal vasculitic changes, an allergic rash along with Raynaud's phenomenon and joint and muscle stiffness. Tender, superficial vessels, granulomatous erosions of the nasal septum and retinal changes should all be looked for. Laboratory investigations may reveal an anaemia which can be due to gastrointestinal blood loss or haemolysis. The while cell count may be reduced, but with a relative increase in lymphocytes and eosinophils. If intravascular coagulation is present then fibrin degradation products are increased. Immunoglobulin levels are raised, often with a reduction in complement levels. Rheumatoid factor and DNA may be isolated. Specific renal investigations may reveal a reduction in the filtration rate and a significant proteinuria. Radiology of the chest may demonstrate pulmonary involvement with or without pleural effusions.

Treatment generally follows a standard approach that involves the use of steroids, cyclophosphamide and azathioprine in the first instance. If intravascular coagulation predominates then anticoagulants and the use of antiplatelet drugs such as aspirin and dipyridamole may prove beneficial. The removal of circulating immune complexes by plasmapheresis and by sustaining prostacyclin activity with Indocid or Ticlopodin is still being assessed. An outline of the clinical entities will now be presented.

Systemic lupus erythematosus (SLE)

This multisystem disease affects middle-aged women more than men. The precise cause of the vascular damage is uncertain, but antibodies are raised against nuclear material, and it is the deposition of antibody-antigen complex within the vessel walls that produces the local damage.

At least 50 per cent of the patients have some degree of renal involvement which in terms of glomerular pathology is manifest in the majority as a proliferative lesion with crescent formation; a few patients exhibit only a focal proliferation, and in a few there is thickening of the basement membrane only.

Early descriptions suggested that blue-staining nuclear fragments (haematoxylin bodies) or thickened capillary loops (the wire loop lesion) were common and pathognomonic. Extended studies have shown that no histological pattern is unique. The proliferative lesions are associated with haematuria, proteinuria and hypertension and often rapidly deteriorating renal function, while heavy proteinuria – often to nephrotic levels – is associated more commonly with a membranous lesion.

Many other systems are involved. Skin rashes which are photosensitive, often affecting the face in a butterfly distribution, are present during periods of activity, while some patients exhibit a discoid lesion. Arthritis, pericarditis, myocarditis and pleural infiltrates with effusions are more serious manifestations, but perhaps the most serious is central nervous system involvement in the form of a transverse myelitis or diffuse cerebral damage.

Patients are often anaemic with a positive Coomb's test, leucopenic and have a raised sedimentation rate. Immunological tests reveal a positive antinuclear factor and low complement levels, and antibody can be detected against DNA.

Treatment is along the lines previously described to improve the prognosis, but death from renal and cerebral involvement is still common. SLE is not a contraindication to renal transplantation as it rarely affects the transplant, a factor which just adds to the aetiological mystery.

Polyarteritis nodosa (PAN)

Here vessels of a larger diameter are involved, and with vessel wall necrosis small aneurysms develop. Men are predominantly affected, and only 25 per cent exhibit renal involvement.

The arcuate and interlobar vessels are damaged by fibrinoid necrosis, with aneurysmal formation and obliteration of the lumen, causing distal ischaemia. These lesions can only be detected by angiography, while a renal biopsy will reveal in the majority of patients a hypercellular lesion with microthrombi in the glomerular capillary loops. Once again heart and lungs are involved.

If intestinal vessels are damaged then abdominal pain and bloody diarrhoea are clinical manifestations. Hypertension and renal involvement may produce severe renal failure, but the time taken to reach this stage varies from patient to patient.

Wegener's granulomatosis

This condition is similar to PAN, with smaller vessels and veins being involved; this produces the characteristic granulomatous lesion which can erode the nasal septum and damage the lung parenchyma.

Patients complain of a bloody nasal discharge, haemoptysis, dyspnoea and pleuritic pain. Careful nasal examination often reveals the characteristic lesion, and if it is suspected a specialist ENT examination is helpful. Chest X-ray demonstrates pulmonary infiltration and occasionally cavitating lesions.

There is considerable overlap with PAN in terms of organ involvement, and the kidney is affected by a proliferative necrotizing glomerulonephritis in over 80 per cent of patients.

The response to treatment is better than in most other vasculitic problems.

Systemic sclerosis

Once again many organs are involved, but characteristically the skin becomes thick and inelastic – changes which are most noticeable in the hands and face. There are numerous telangiectases and Raynaud's phenomenon is a prominent feature.

Connective tissue is generally involved, with painful joints, muscle wasting, abdominal pain and malabsorption. Pulmonary fibrosis can lead to respiratory difficulty. This pulmonary involvement involves approximately 30 per cent of the patient group, while renal involvement is present in over half the patients.

Intralobular vessels are narrowed and often occluded by an intimal proliferation – the cells characteristically are full of a blue-staining mucoid-like material.

These changes predominate in the cortex and it is no surprise that this ischaemia produces severe hypertension which is difficult to treat. Powerful hypotensive agents are required, and on occasions a bilateral nephrectomy has to be performed before blood pressure control is achieved. Proliferative glomerulonephritis is often present, and this produces haematuria and mild proteinuria. The outcome of treatment is unpredictable.

Henoch–Schönlein purpura

This vasculitic process affects mainly children, but young adults may be similarly afflicted. Four clinical features predominate:

(1) Raised purpuric lesions on the extensor surfaces of limbs and buttocks, in the presence of a normal platelet count, is a non-thrombocytopenic purpura that may respond to topical steroids or dapsone.
(2) Vessels of the alimentary tract may be involved, producing abdominal pain and haemorrhage. Surgery is often indicated.
(3) There may be painful inflammation of knees and ankles.
(4) There may be proteinuria, haematuria and progressive renal failure owing to inflammation of the glomerular vessels. Several histological changes from the renal biopsy have been reported, ranging from the involvement of the occasional glomerulus with basement membrane thickening, to a proliferative lesion and widespread glomerular sclerosis. The former lesion is often associated with heavy proteinuria, while the proliferative lesions are associated with progressive renal failure. Once again the response to treatment varies and the value of plasmapheresis is still uncertain.

This brief summary is sufficient to show that there is considerable overlap in presentation of the various syndromes that seem to share antigen–antibody complex-mediated damage to the vessel walls. The response to treatment varies considerably, and if end-stage renal failure is reached the involvement of other systems is often so severe that dialysis and transplantation are inappropriate. However, it has been undertaken successfully in some patients, and so each patient needs to be assessed on his or her own merits.

Amyloid deposition

Histologically, amyloid is an amorphous eosinophilic material that has other staining characteristics, namely it will stain with congo red and exhibit green birefringence in polarized light. It is deposited in many organs and can occur as a primary condition or secondary to chronic suppuration, rheumatoid arthritis or in association with multiple myeloma and familial Mediterranean fever.

The chemical composition of amyloid is complex and is the subject of continuing research. Two main components, A and B, have been isolated, but as yet there is no therapeutic implication associated with these chemical differences.

Apart from renal involvement, myocardial infiltration may cause cardiac failure, and occlusion of nutrient vessels to the major nerves leads to a peripheral neuropathy. General organ infiltration produces an enlargement of liver and spleen without any constitutional upset.

In the kidney, amyloid deposition starts in the interlobular arteries. The thickening of the glomerular arterioles and finally involvement of the capillary loops leads to progressive renal failure. As the walls of the capillaries become thickened, amyloid can mimic membranous glomerulonephritis; special stains and polarized light, and electron microscopy which can demonstrate the amyloid fibrils, are essential to make an accurate diagnosis.

These changes produce proteinuria, the commonest form of presentation. The protein loss can reach 10–20 g/24 hours, producing the nephrotic syndrome. Occlusion of the glomerular tufts impairs renal function which can suddenly further deteriorate as renal vein thrombosis is a common complication. Infiltration of the peritubular vessels can produce a range of tubular defects.

If amyloid is secondary to chronic sepsis its eradication may prevent further deposition, but other forms do not respond to therapy, with patients dying of cardiac or renal failure. Recent therapeutic attempts with steroids, melphalan, penicillamine and most recently dimethylsulphoxide have all proved fruitless.

If no other organ is involved then dialysis and transplantation can be successful, but amyloid recurrence within a renal transplant has been reported.

Multiple myeloma

When plasma cells in the bone marrow increase and produce increased levels of immunoglobulins (the majority producing IgG with a few IgA and IgD), renal involvement is responsible for some of the clinical problems. As well as increased levels of intact IgG there are circulating light and heavy chain fragments; these are freely filtered at the glomerulus and precipitate to form dense casts within the tubular lumen. The presence of casts stimulates a local tubular cellular reaction. These casts produce obstruction which, if permanent, can produce renal failure. Dehydration will promote cast deposition and obstruction, and therefore this should be avoided if at all possible. Certainly a patient being prepared for an IVU should not be subjected to fluid deprivation. It is thought that some of the smaller immunoglobulin fragments are reabsorbed into the tubular cells where they produce multiple tubular defects of a Fanconi type.

A further reason for loss of concentrating ability and tubular damage is the presence of a raised serum calcium produced by local bone destruction by the plasma cells. Parenchymal infection can increase the renal damage and in about 10 per cent of patients amyloid deposition occurs. These changes, along with (occasionally) a dense infiltration of plasma cells, can be detected by a renal biopsy.

Renal size has been mentioned as an important factor in assessing patients with renal failure. It is important to note that with myeloma the kidneys are enlarged. The other important causes are obstruction and infiltration with amyloid.

Other clinical features include general malaise associated with concurrent anaemia and bone pain. Diagnostic features include the detection in plasma and urine of immunoglobulins by electrophoresis, and radiologically erosions in the cortex of long bones. A bone marrow aspiration may reveal an increase in plasma cells but, as they have a patchy distribution throughout the marrow, the biopsy may not be diagnostic.

With the increased level of circulating gammaglobulin blood viscosity may be increased, a factor which predisposes to intravascular coagulation. A measurement of the blood viscosity is an important factor in the initial assessment of the patient and in following the progress of therapy.

Treatment is often successful and the use of cytotoxic agents such as melphalan have improved the prognosis. Patients should be well hydrated at all times, and alkalinization may prevent cast formation within the kidney. With nuclear destruction by cytotoxic agents there follows an increased production of uric acid, which may also produce renal damage; allopurinol, which inhibits uric acid synthesis, is often added to the treatment regimen. Hypercalcaemic damage is prevented by ensuring adequate hydration and by the use of steroids.

Gout

The relationship between renal damage and a raised uric acid, with or without joint involvement, is not clear. There is no doubt that, in patients with long-standing joint involvement, uric acid crystals can be demonstrated histologically within the tubules. Patients often complain of polyuria, suggesting a deficit in concentrating ability. However these changes are not sufficient to cause renal impairment to a degree which limits life expectancy.

Two circumstances, however, are important:

(1) The sudden rise in uric acid associated with the cytotoxic treatment of malignancy can lead to an increased filtered load. If dehydration is associated, then intraluminal crystal formation may lead to obstruction. Allopurinol, which limits uric acid production, along with alkalinization of the urine to prevent crystal deposition, are important adjuncts to aggressive chemotherapy.

(2) Uric acid calculi represent one-fifth of all renal stones and may cause obstruction and renal damage. These stones are not radio-opaque and are often only detected during an IVU or antegrade or retrograde examination. Treatment is along similar lines.

Sarcoid lesions

Rarely the kidney can be involved directly by a granulomatous lesion, and on occasions a membranous glomerulonephritis seems to be an associated finding. More commonly tubular defects in the form of impaired concentrating and acidification ability are reported.

This tubular damage may be due directly to the sarcoid lesion itself, or it may be associated with a raised serum calcium produced by increased sensitivity to vitamin D.

Pregnancy

The changes that occur in renal function during a normal pregnancy are important. When considering the relationship between renal disease and pregnancy, two general areas have to be discussed: first the effect of pregnancy on renal function, and secondly the converse, namely the influence that impaired renal function will have upon the pregnancy itself.

The effect of pregnancy on renal function

Normal physiological changes

During the first and second trimester there are approximately 50 per cent increases in the renal blood flow and glomerular filtration rate; during the third trimester these return towards normal, and are completely normal after delivery. There is general sodium and water retention, producing expansion of the plasma volume by as much as 50 per cent. Increased levels of circulating angiotensin II and catecholamines clearly play a part in these changes.

The blood pressure falls during the first trimester and then gradually returns towards normal at term. Minimal proteinuria, possibly as a result of inferior vena caval obstruction and a rise in renal vein pressures, does occur, but again after delivery there is no excessive protein loss.

Abnormal changes

With the development of pre-eclampsia there is excessive sodium and water retention, proteinuria and hypertension. These changes are more common in primigravid women and are often associated with fetal abnormalities, hydatidiform mole or pre-existing renal disease.

Renal biopsies show that there is no proliferation of the glomerular cells, but rather a swelling of the endothelial and mesangial cells which gradually obliterate the glomerular space. The interlobular and glomerular arterioles have reduplication of their elastic lamina and some cellular proliferation.

Increased levels of endotoxins, angiotensin, excessive fibrinolysis and immune mechanisms have all been blamed, but no clear aetiological picture has emerged. With bed rest, control of hypertension and careful monitoring of fetal and placental function the outcome for mother and fetus is generally good, without any persistent renal damage.

More serious damage occurs in the form of bilateral cortical necrosis, often associated with concealed antepartum haemorrhage. The area of necrosis is patchy and the chance of long-term recovery with adequate renal function is good.

Postpartum renal failure rarely occurs. When it does it presents in a similar fashion to the haemolytic uraemic syndrome, but the aetiology is not clear.

The effect of pre-existing renal disease on pregnancy

Patients with previous renal disease, especially associated with some degree of functional impairment, are more likely to develop pre-eclampsia and have poor placental function associated with reduced fetal growth. Close liaison between the renal physician and obstetrician is essential.

Modern techniques of ultrasound and hormonal assay, close monitoring of renal and placental function, coupled with an index of fetal growth, are important measurements that should be repeated throughout pregnancy. Rest and control of blood pressure are still the central features of management, and induction of labour coupled with skilful care of the newborn have allowed some women to achieve success when in the past the thought of pregnancy would not have been even considered.

Not all renal lesions will be untouched by pregnancy. Active glomerulonephritis, especially related to SLE and PAN, may relapse, and in some patients an active glomerulonephritis develops during pregnancy for the first time. In this group the prognosis for the fetus is not good. Patients with congenital abnormalities of the lower tract and polycystic kidneys are prone to develop severe infection which may result in permanent loss of renal function. An established functioning transplant should not create problems, but once again meticulous joint care is essential.

16

Pharmacology

Principles

The aim of drug treatment is to liberate free drug into the circulation where it can be delivered to the receptor site of the target organ and there exert its effect. Routes of adminstration are many: rapid intravenous injection produces immediately detectable blood levels; with oral administration there is a delay while absorption takes place, and peak blood levels are reached approximately 40–60 minutes after ingestion.

Many factors control gastrointestinal absorption, from gut motility to the timing of the previous meal. The drug enters the portal system and passes through the liver. Metabolism takes place, and it is often the metabolite that is the active compound.

Once in the blood, free drug is bound to tissue, enters cells (especially if the drug is fat soluble) and is bound to plasma proteins. Tissue binding may remove over 90 per cent of the drug during the first circulation through the body: for example, 80 per cent of intravenous propranolol is bound to lung parenchyma. Binding to plasma protein is important as this is reversible and the bound drug acts as a reservoir to maintain circulating levels (Fig. 16.1).

Apart from volatile anaesthetic agents (which can be excreted via the lungs), the prime routes of excretion of drugs are via the liver (the drug or its metabolites being eliminated in the bile) or via the kidneys. Drugs can be cleared by the kidney either by glomerular filtration or tubular secretion. The latter can take the form of active secretion or passive non-ionic diffusion, a process often governed by the pH of the tubular fluid. (A common example of pH-dependent diffusion is of the salicylates, which diffuse very readily into an alkaline medium: hence the use of a forced alkaline diuresis in the management of an overdose.) It is clear that the plasma level is the result of many factors.

If serial measurements are taken after administration of a single dose, the rate of disappearance can be expressed as the *half-life*, which is the time taken for the plasma level to fall by 50 per cent, assuming that the decay from the bloodstream is exponential. This value gives a good index of the rate of overall clearance. It can range from minutes to days.

This approach, however, is only half the story as in some cases the drug is clearly exerting a biological effect at a time when no free drug can be detected in

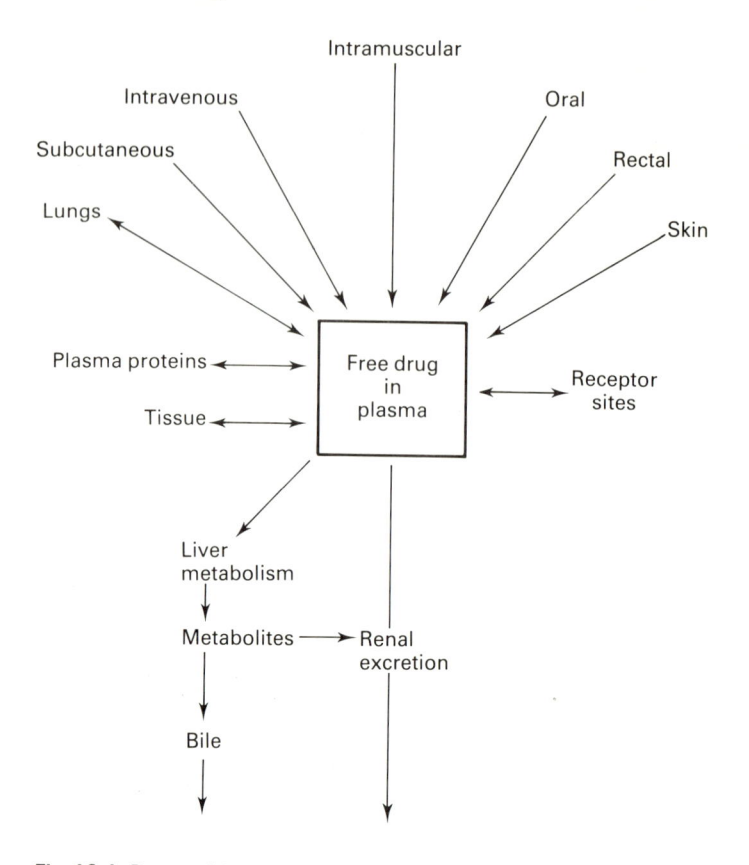

Fig. 16.1 Routes of drug administration, and the potential fate of free drug in the plasma.

the plasma, i.e. the biological half-life is longer than the chemical half-life. One explanation is that drugs reach the receptor sites and remain active there despite elimination of free drug from the circulation. Clearly the duration of the biological effect is important clinically, but it is often difficult to assess with accuracy in routine practice.

This normal sequence of events is altered in several ways when drugs are used in the presence of renal failure. The plasma half-life is prolonged when filtration is a major route of drug elimination, and no alternative biliary route is available (e.g. with the aminoglycosides and digoxin). Protein binding may be reduced, resulting in an increase in the circulating level to possibly toxic concentration. Other drugs given simultaneously may have a greater affinity for the plasma protein sites, thus displacing the drugs in question. The displacement of warfarin by other drugs is well known, making anticoagulation control difficult. Drug metabolism may be altered in renal failure (e.g. the metabolism of vitamin D by the kidney is decreased in renal failure, whereas that of insulin appears to be enhanced). These changes may mean that after a normal loading dose the amount of each subsequent dose and the frequency of administration may need to be drastically reduced.

Reference to a standard pharmacology text and to the review papers that are produced periodically covering the new therapeutic agents will give the appropriate details. There is no excuse for the clinician not to be aware of these data when prescribing, and to be familiar with the possible side-effects of therapy, some of which may produce renal damage.

Nephrotoxicity

There are several reasons why the kidney is susceptible to drug damage. Three most important of those reasons are:

(1) the kidney has a rich blood supply;
(2) the medulla is hyperosmotic and drugs may be concentrated in this region;
(3) the kidney is prone to immunological damage which may be triggered by drug administration.

Common and serious problems are encountered when drugs that are potentially directly nephrotoxic lead to acute renal failure. If the condition is spotted early and the drug withdrawn, then there is a good chance of recovery of renal function; but supportive dialysis may be required. The list of such drugs is long, and other factors are often present. Commonly the aminoglycosides are blamed for producing acute renal failure, but sepsis and the associated hypotension demanding the use of such powerful drugs are often major contributory factors. The common offenders, each with a brief note, are listed in Table 16.1.

Manifestations other than acute renal failure

A systemic lupus-like syndrome with a positive antinuclear factor in the serum can be produced by hydralazine, isoniazid, phenytoin, penicillamine and phenylbutazone.

The nephrotic syndrome, often due to a membranous lesion, can occur with penicillamine, tolbutamide, probenecid, troxidone and gold.

Retroperitoneal fibrosis is often idiopathic, but in some cases it can be related to the administration of methysergide or ergotamine.

Analgesic nephropathy is associated with the ingestion over long periods of phenacetin. Other analgesics have been blamed, but the evidence is not so convincing. Tubular damage with loss of acidification and concentration are the early changes. Interstitial nephritis and papillary necrosis lead to progressive loss of filtration, and in some cases acute loss of function may be associated with obstruction following the shedding of a papilla. Some improvement can be achieved when the drug is stopped. Transitional cell tumours of the renal pelvis, ureter and bladder occur more commonly in this group.

Table 16.1 Side-effects of some common drugs

Aminoglycosides	These drugs are ototoxic, producing giddiness which often persists after renal function has returned. Frequent monitoring of the blood level and appropriate reduction of dose and frequency is essential. Levels should be measured before a dose is given, giving the trough level, and after administration, giving the peak value; both are important readings on which to judge further drug administration.
Sulphonamides	Intratubular crystal aggregation may cause obstruction which can be cleared by alkali and fluid administration. Vasculitic damage has also been reported.
Cephalosporins	Acute tubular damage – less frequent with the new generation of compounds.
Polymyxin	Also neurotoxic.
Rifampicin	Tubular damage and interstitial nephritis.
Amphotericin	Predominantly produces tubular damage, but acute vasoconstriction may be responsible for rapid reductions in glomerular filtration rate which can return rapidly to normal once the drug has been discontinued.
Cyclosporin-A	Used as an antirejection agent; it can also cause vascular damage.
Phenindione	Allergic glomerulonephritis.
Cisplatin	A cytotoxic drug which is also nephrotoxic.
General anaesthetic agents	Mainly methoxyflurane – produces tubular damage and, as it is metabolised to oxalic acid, crystal deposition within the kidney may cause acute renal failure. This, however, is rare.
Tetracycline	Antianabolic and in some cases directly nephrotoxic.
Radiographic contrast	Strictly not a drug, but mentioned here as reports of nephrotoxicity following intra-arterial injection have been made. Dehydration should be avoided in patients with impaired renal function, and the use of isotonic constrast media may limit renal damage.

17
Cancer of the genitourinary tract

Haematuria

Physiological blood loss

The urinary tract normally excretes 40,000 red blood cells per hour (20,000 in children). This physiological loss shows diurnal variation and is increased, sometimes markedly, during all forms of physical exercise. Until recently the screening method for microscopic haematuria ('stick test') was too insensitive to pick up so small a number of cells. As direct microscopy of centrifuged urine was usually only performed for some clinical indication, it was reasonable to say that symptomless microscopic haematuria was clinically significant.

The new urine dip sticks (e.g. N-Multistix, Ames Ltd) are so sensitive and so widely used that large numbers of symptomless patients with minimal microscopic haematuria are being found. Present indications are that there is very little wrong with these patients and investigations should be limited.

Apart from this physiological blood loss, the normal urinary tract does not bleed. All patients presenting with haematuria require investigation.

Pathological blood loss

Any part of the urinary tract may bleed. Lesions in the kidneys, ureters or bladder usually produce blood fully mixed with urine, often with clots. Red cells from the renal parenchyma are often distorted by passage through the tubules or are stuck together as casts of the renal tubules.

'String-like' clots have usually come from upper tract bleeding, the clots being formed in the ureter. Bleeding from the prostate is sometimes only apparent at the beginning of voiding. Urethral lesions may only bleed at the end of voiding, or the bleeding may be spontaneous and unassociated with voiding.

Very many lesions present with bleeding, but knowledge of the pathophysiology allows logical investigation.

Vascular problems

Hypertension may push blood through the glomeruli by increased filtration pressure, or may damage the glomeruli which then allow red cell leakage. In either case, hypertension associated with microscopic haematuria carries a poor prognosis.

Abnormal capillaries, as in scurvy, allow spontaneous bleeding at many sites. Clotting defects (such as haemophilia or anticoagulant therapy) do not usually cause bleeding from a normal urinary tract.

Inflammatory lesions

An inflammatory process will cause hyperaemia and bleeding. Usually the bleeding is accompanied by symptoms of inflammation such as voiding frequency and dysuria. Some chronic inflammatory diseases, particularly tuberculosis, cause painless haematuria.

Urinary tract stones cause inflammation through local trauma. Bleeding is usually microscopic but can be gross.

Trauma

Any injury, particularly to the kidney, can produce haematuria which may go on for several days or weeks. Healing of renal injuries may be complicated by formation of an arteriovenous fistula which is itself a source of bleeding. If bleeding is greater than expected from the severity of the trauma, an underlying abnormality should be suspected. Congenital renal lesions, such as hydronephrosis, are often unmasked in this way.

Neoplasms

All neoplasms, especially malignant ones, are supplied by thin-walled, fragile vessels which allow spontaneous bleeding. This is the single commonest cause of haematuria in the Western world.

Investigation of haematuria

All patients presenting with haematuria must be fully investigated, but the emphasis will vary according to their age.

Patients over 40 years

Patients over 40 years with haematuria are considered to have cancer unless proved otherwise. Minimum investigation consists of urine microscopy and culture; urine cytology (providing a skilled cytologist is available); intravenous urography; cystoscopy and bimanual examination under anaesthetic. The physical examination or the results of special investigations may suggest additional procedures. If no cause for haematuria is found immediately, the patient must be kept under review.

Patients from 16 to 39 years

Patients in this age group are very much less likely to have cancer. The commonest cause of haematuria is infection, with stones and glomerulonephritis also important. Minimum investigation includes measurement of blood pressure; urine microscopy and culture; urine cytology (if available); and a plain abdominal X-ray for stones. The number of possible diagnoses is so large that further investigation must proceed according to clinical suspicion.

In sexually active women, haematuria associated with recurrent, proven, bacterial cystitis requires no further investigation except under the circumstances set out in Chapter 9. In men, recurrent cystitis is nearly always caused by chronic bacterial prostatitis. Abnormalities of renal function such as hypertension, proteinuria or abnormal electrolytes, urea or creatinine, indicate glomerulonephritis. Phase contrast microscopy of urinary red blood cells can distinguish those of intrarenal as opposed to collecting system origin.

If these simple, non-invasive investigations give no clue to the origin of haematuria, intravenous urogram and cystoscopy should be performed. After all of this a few cases remain with persistent, and often heavy, haematuria from an unknown source. It is helpful to examine the patient and perform cystoscopy while he is actually bleeding: at least the organ responsible may be identified so that further investigation can be planned.

Children

Haematuria in children is very rarely from a 'surgical' cause. Although the same preliminary investigations as for young adults are reasonable (omitting urine cytology), further endeavour should be directed at the kidney. Intravenous urography is of little use, especially in the very young. Glomerulonephritis is the commonest cause.

Cancer of the kidney

There are two main cancers of the kidney. One arises from the transitional epithelium of the renal collecting system and will be considered under urothelial cancer. The other one is renal cell cancer.

Renal cell cancer has had various names since it was first described over 100 years ago. It has borne the eponym of its discoverer, Grawitz. It has been called 'clear cell tumour' (from the appearance of the commonest cell type) and hypernephroma. These names have caused much confusion and should not be used. Renal cell, renal parenchymal or renal tubular cell carcinoma, or renal adenocarcinoma, are all acceptable titles. Renal cell carcinoma is the most commonly used.

Incidence and aetiology

Renal cell carcinoma accounts for about 3 per cent of cancer deaths in England and Wales. For unknown reasons it is commoner in Scotland, New Zealand, Norway and Denmark; and less common in Ireland, Italy, Spain, Venezuela and, especially, Japan. It is about twice as common in men as in women.

No definite causes have been found. In experimental animals a very wide range of carcinogenic agents have been found, but none is relevant in man.

Pathology

Renal cell cancer is an adenocarcinoma arising in the proximal convoluted tubules or, occasionally, in the ducts of Bellini. The cells show a range of differentiation and have been arbitrarily divided into well, moderately and poorly differentiated groups which loosely correlate with prognosis.

Symptomless 'adenomas' are a common post-mortem finding. Histologically they are indistinguishable from carcinomas. Only 3 per cent of those under 3 cm in diameter have metastases. If a small 'adenoma' is found incidentally in a patient it should be treated as cancer and removed.

Renal cell carcinoma spreads locally through the parenchyma until it bursts out into the perinephric fat. In a few cases it invades adjacent structures such as psoas muscle, tail of pancreas, splenic flexure (on the left), duodenum or hepatic flexure (on the right). The ipsilateral adrenal is involved in 20 per cent of cases, probably by venous spread. Invasion of the renal collecting system occurs relatively late, so that haematuria, as a presentation, is likely to indicate advanced disease.

The pattern of lymph node spread is curious. Presumably the local hilar nodes are the first site, yet sometimes distant nodal metastases are found without any in the local nodes.

Distant metastases can be found almost anywhere but are commonest in lung, bone and liver. Considering the very long interval that may occur between nephrectomy and the appearances of overt metastases, it is possible that microscopic metastases are very common and remain 'dormant' until circumstances are right for rapid growth.

Presentation

Three-quarters of patients present with one or more of the so called 'classic triad' of renal pain, haematuria and loin mass (Table 17.1). Ten per cent are chance findings, either with metastases or during examinations for other reasons. A few left-sided cancers present with a varicocele, though the reason is unknown and it does not appear to be due to venous involvement by tumour:

Table 17.1 Presentations of renal cell carcinoma

	(%)
'Classic triad'	2
Haematuria alone	40
Pain alone	10
Mass alone	2
2 of triad	25
Constitutional symptoms	10
Varicocele	1
Other	10

Cancer of the kidney   175

Table 17.2 Systemic manifestations of renal adenocarcinoma

Clinical features	Laboratory features	Associations
(a) *Endocrine:*		
Hypercalcaemia	Raised serum calcium, low or normal phosphate	
Erythrocytosis	Raised red cell count and plasma erythropoietin; other blood elements normal; normal arterial oxygen tension	No splenomegaly
Hypertension	Rarely raised renal vein renin	Poor prognosis
Others (very rare)	Raised: gonadotrophins placental lactogens enteroglucagon insulin ADH prostaglandins	Diagnostic curiosities
(b) *Biochemical:*		
Hepatosplenomegaly	Abnormal liver function tests	Fever, weight loss, anaemia; no liver metastases
(c) *Non-specific:*		
Pyrexia	Non-white cell pyrogen	
Anaemia	Normochromic, normocytic	
Amyloidosis		Nephrotic syndrome (rare)
Non-metastatic neuromyopathy		

presumably there is a haemodynamic disturbance. It should be remembered that the left spermatic vein drains into the left renal vein. The remainder present with a variety of constitutional syndromes (Table 17.2). Renal carcinomas may produce several enzymes or hormones in up to 30 per cent of cases. They may be detected by appropriate tests, and they are important tumour markers since they are usually produced by the metastases as well as the primary. In 10 per cent of cases they are produced in sufficient quantities to give rise to recognizable syndromes. When this occurs the cancers may be diagnosed relatively earlier in their natural history.

Investigation

Whatever the presentation, the first definitive investigation for most patients is an intravenous urogram. A renal cell carcinoma is indicated by a mass of non-functioning parenchyma which distorts the outline of the kidney and the calyces. This finding is known in urological jargon as a 'space occupying lesion' (Fig. 17.1). The differential diagnosis is from renal cysts: on IVU these are seen as smooth, round masses which displace rather than distort the collecting system. Malignant renal cysts are extremely rare. Ultrasound examination will

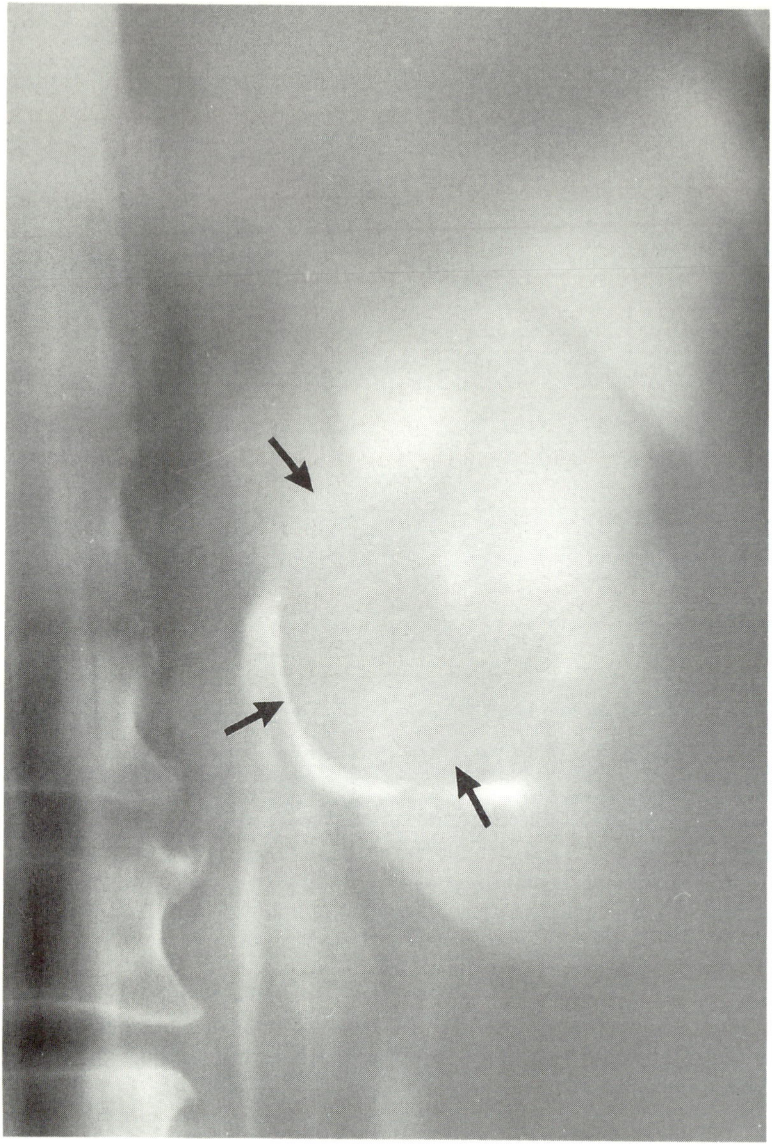

176 *Cancer of the genitourinary tract*

Fig. 17.1 Tomogram of the IVU of a left kidney, showing a mass in the middle displacing the renal pelvis and obstructing the upper pole calyx.

distinguish between solid lesions which are neoplasms (Fig. 17.2), and smooth, fluid-filled lesions which are cysts. If there is still doubt about the diagnosis, the mass can be needled under ultrasound control to drain the fluid and to get cells for cytological examination.

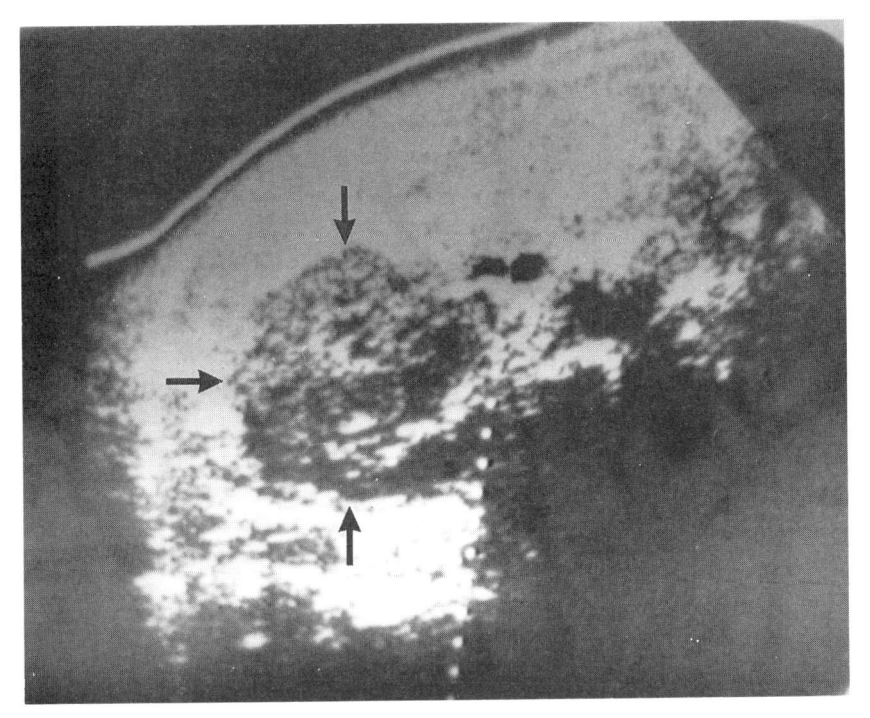

Fig. 17.2 Ultrasound picture of a renal mass with many (white) echoes indicating its solid nature.

Before deciding on treatment, staging of the disease is essential. The best single investigation is abdominal ultrasound which shows the size of local tumour, spread into the renal vein or inferior vena cava, size of the local lymph nodes and presence of liver metastases. Abdominal and thoracic computerized axial tomography may be necessary in some cases. Pulmonary metastases, the commonest site, are seen on chest X-ray or whole-lung tomography. Venacavography is indicated to define the extent of caval involvement.

The search for the abnormalities listed in Table 17.2 depends on the facilities available. Full blood count, ESR, serum calcium, phosphate and liver enzymes are the minimum. If there are no metastases any abnormal parameters should become normal after nephrectomy. Subsequent development of metastases will make them abnormal again.

Treatment

The only possible cure for renal cell cancer is surgical removal. Radiotherapy and chemotherapy have little to offer. If there are no distant metastases the kidney should be removed along with perinephric fascia, perinephric fat and adrenal gland.

Venous involvement is *not* a contraindication to nephrectomy: the tumour should be removed from the vein, if necessary opening the IVC or even the right atrium. A solitary pulmonary metastasis can also be removed, usually at a second operation.

Nephrectomy should not be performed in the presence of multiple metastases unless there are severe local symptoms which cannot be controlled in any other way. It does not lengthen life. It has often been suggested that the metastases will regress if the primary is removed, but this is an extremely rare event: the incidence of spontaneous regression is less than the operative mortality. In any event, spontaneous regression is not a cure, only a temporary radiological improvement.

Metastatic disease should be treated symptomatically. Painful bone metastases respond to local radiotherapy. About 10 per cent of cases will respond to oral medroxy-progesterone (100 mg t.d.s.).

Prognosis

Twenty-five per cent of patients have metastases at presentation or develop them soon after nephrectomy and are dead within a year. In the remainder prognosis is related to stage and, to a lesser extent, the grade of tumour. Carcinoma apparently confined to the kidney has a 66 per cent 5-year survival and a 50 per cent 10-year survival. This means that some patients who seem disease-free at 5 years do, in fact, have microscopic metastases which develop and from which they die. Late metastases are common, and examples have been reported up to 20 years after nephrectomy. Obvious local extension of the primary into perinephric fat lowers the 5- and 10-year survival rates to 50 and 35 per cent respectively.

Cancer of the urothelium

Cancer of the epithelial lining of the urinary tract is the most important single 'urological' disease in terms of the time occupied in treatment. The epithelium from the renal collecting ducts to the distal one-sixth of the urethra is transitional cell in origin and peculiarly prone to neoplasia. Once a tumour has appeared in one area it must be assumed that all of the urinary epithelium of that patient is at risk and, for convenience, it is referred to as 'urothelial' cancer. The urinary epithelium can also give rise to adenocarcinomas and squamous carcinomas which will be considered separately.

Incidence and aetiology

Transitional cell carcinoma is the commonest cancer of the urinary tract in the Western world. It is not the commonest cause of death from cancer of the urinary tract because many cases run a relatively benign course. It is commonest in industrialized countries and in the most industrialized areas of those countries. Several specific industries have a particularly high incidence (Table 17.3).

In some cases specific carcinogens have been identified. Although exposure to the carcinogen need only be brief, the latent period before a clinical cancer

Table 17.3 Industrial causes of transitional cell carcinoma of the bladder

(a) *Proven carcinogens:*
Beta-naphthylamine
Other naphthylamines and diazo dyes
Auramine
Magenta

(b) *Industries recognized to have a high rate of bladder carcinoma:*
Coal gas production (especially in the retort shops)
Natural rubber users
Processes involving use or purification of chemical carcinogens

(c) *Occupations with a suspected but unproven risk:*
Rat catching
Printing
Leather working

appears is up to 30 years. It is commoner in smokers, and a smoker exposed to an industrial carcinogen has nearly double the risk of a non-smoker.

Patients with papillary necrosis have a high incidence of intrarenal urothelial carcinoma.

Pathology

The first tumour may appear anywhere in the urinary tract, but in over 90 per cent of cases it is in the bladder. Transitional cell carcinomas have a very wide range of differentiation, staging at presentation and subsequent natural history. The gross appearance ranges from a papillary tumour that arises from the mucosa on a stalk, to a solid and sometimes necrotic mass involving all layers of the muscle wall.

Accurate staging is critical to the management of transitional cell carcinoma and correlates very closely with prognosis. For the bladder it is set out in detail in Table 17.4 and Fig. 17.3.

Three grades of differentiation are recognized — well, moderately and poorly differentiated. Some anaplastic tumours probably arise from the transitional epithelium. Areas of squamous metaplasia are commonly seen but are not of clinical significance. Pure squamous carcinomas of the bladder are rare in the

Table 17.4 Staging of bladder carcinoma using the TNM system: combined surgical and pathological staging of the local tumour (from Union Internationale Contre de Cancer)

pTis	Carcinoma *in situ*
pTa	Papillary, non-invasive tumour
pT1	No tumour beyond the lamina propria
pT2	Invasion of superficial muscle
pT3a	Invasion of deep muscle
pT3b	Extension into perivesical tissue
pT4a	Invasion of the prostate or uterus
pT4b	Invasion of any other pelvic organ or the pelvic side wall

It is important to distinguish between pathological staging (shown here and prefaced by 'p') and the clinical staging shown in Figure 17.3 which is made without knowledge of the histology.

180 Cancer of the genitourinary tract

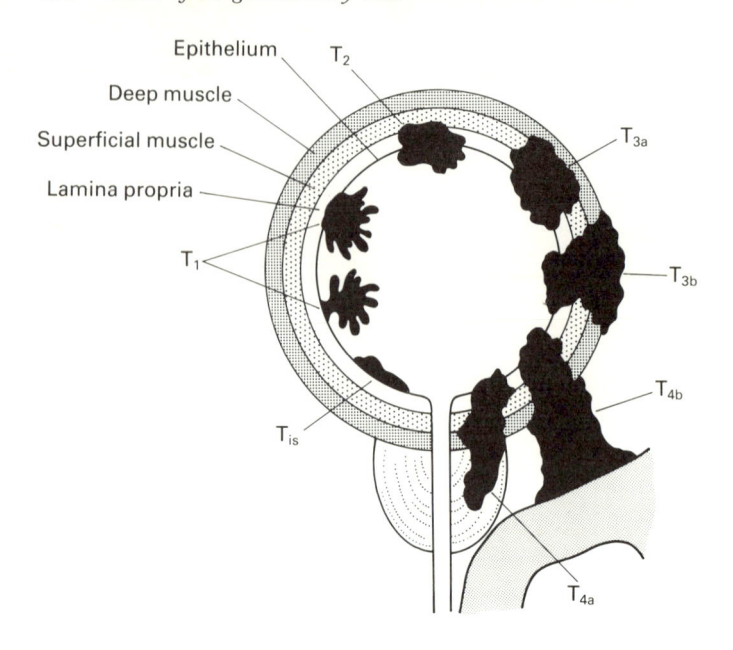

T   Primary tumour
N   Regional lymph nodes
M   Metastases

Fig. 17.3 The *clinical* staging of bladder cancer.

United Kingdom but common in countries with a high incidence of bilharzia. No case of bladder cancer should have definitive management until it has been accurately graded and staged.

Bladder carcinoma, even when very aggressive, remains confined to the pelvis until late in the course of the disease. Tumours confined to the urothelium and lamina propria are loosely referred to as 'non-invasive' or 'superficial' and have a good prognosis. Tumours invading through the bladder muscle and into adjacent pelvic structures are, obviously, 'invasive'.

Ten per cent of patients with muscle invasion have lymph node involvement detectable on lymphangiography at presentation.

Remote metastases occur in lung, liver and bones in about equal proportions. However, they are detectable in less than 5 per cent of subjects on conventional imaging at presentation.

As 60 per cent of patients with muscle invasion will ultimately die of their cancer in spite of radical local treatment, it is probable that micrometastases are present but are undetectable.

Natural history (modified by treatment)

About 70 per cent of bladder cancers are 'superficial' and well or moderately differentiated. There may be single or multiple tumours. They should receive

Table 17.5 Adverse prognostic factors in transitional cell carcinoma of the bladder

History	Exposure to industrial carcinogens
	Smoking
	Delay in diagnosis
Examination	Multiple tumours
	Frequent recurrences
Pathological	High grade
	Dysplasia or carcinoma *in situ* remote from the main tumour

local treatment. Regular cystoscopy will establish a pattern of recurrent local tumours which are almost always 'downstream' of the original and of the same histology. Seventy-five per cent of cases should be maintained on local treatment for bladder recurrences (if any). Twenty-five per cent will progress in stage or grade or will prove impossible to control by local means; they will require radical treatment. The skill in managing superficial bladder cancers lies not only in meticulous cystoscopic resection techniques, but also in recognizing those cases which require more radical treatment before they become incurable. Even the most innocent looking tumour may metastasize and it is not for nothing that all are called 'carcinomas'. The adverse prognostic factors are shown in Table 17.5.

The 30 per cent of cases who have muscle invasion from presentation have demonstrated the aggressive nature of the disease from the start. Without radical treatment, it will progress locally, causing unpleasant bladder and pelvic, and ultimately distant, symptoms. One of the consequences of the late distant spread of this disease is that the local symptoms occur long before metastatic disease causes death. Early death from local disease usually only occurs if both ureters become obstructed.

Carcinoma *in situ*

A special mention must be made of carcinoma *in situ*: a condition which in the bladder has caused much confusion.

Carcinoma *in situ* is defined as a malignant change in transitional epithelium without a visible tumour. Cytologically the cells are poorly differentiated, and they exfoliate freely into the urine where they can be found in voided specimens. Usually the change is very widespread or total. In the urinary tract it is a very ominous finding and implies that extensive and aggressive malignant change has already occurred.

Clinically, the following two completely different types of carcinoma *in situ* exist.

Malignant cystitis

Patients present *de novo* with carcinoma *in situ*. It occurs almost exclusively in men. Cytology is positive. On cystoscopy the bladder usually looks inflamed but may appear normal. There is no visible tumour, but histology shows generalized carcinoma *in situ*. Without treatment this condition progresses within 5 years to aggressive, invasive cancer.

Tumour and carcinoma *in situ*

In the early 1950s it was noticed that in some cystectomy specimens, grossly normal mucosa, remote from the obvious tumour, had microscopic carcinoma *in situ*. Modern assessment of any case of bladder carcinoma must now include biopsy of several areas of apparently normal mucosa. The finding of carcinoma *in situ*, in a bladder with a tumour of any local stage, implies a poor prognosis.

Presentation

Painless haematuria is the classic presentation of bladder carcinoma. It is commoner in men than in women. It is rare before 40 years old but can occur as young as 12 years. Other local bladder symptoms can herald the disease, and unexpected urinary tract infection in an older patient should always raise the possibility: 45 per cent of cases of invasive bladder carcinoma have infected urine.

In 'malignant cystitis' patients have severe and unremitting symptoms of cystitis without infection. The symptoms cause considerable anxiety and agitation and, in the past, patients have been sent to mental hospitals. Urine cytology or bladder biopsy will reveal the right diagnosis.

Very occasionally a patient will present with advanced local disease which has caused renal failure (from bilateral ureteric obstruction) or rectal symptoms. Presentation from remote metastases is rare.

Investigation

The diagnosis can be made from urinary cytology, intravenous urogram (Fig. 17.4) and cystoscopy. All three are essential. It cannot be said too often that all adult patients with painless haematuria must undergo cystoscopy: many patients have bladder cancer despite normal urograms and negative cytology.

Diagnostic cystoscopy should be performed under general anaesthesia deep enough to relax the abdominal wall muscles. In men the cystoscope should be introduced under direct vision so that the urethra can be inspected. After careful inspection, representative biopsies of tumours, suspicious areas and normal mucosa are taken. Small tumours are cauterized and larger ones resected. A careful bimanual examination of the pelvis is done before and after resection of tumour: the clinical distinction between T1, T2, T3 and T4 tumours is made at this examination (Fig. 17.3). 'Non-invasive' tumours need no further investigation unless they are poorly differentiated. 'Invasive tumours' and poorly differentiated tumours are staged by lymphangiography and/or computerized axial tomography for lymph node involvement. Investigation for distant metastases is unrewarding: bone scan, liver scan and even routine chest X-ray seldom pick up metastases in bladder cancer unless they are large enough to be clinically obvious. Although most lung metastases are, themselves, asymptomatic, they

Cancer of the urothelium 183

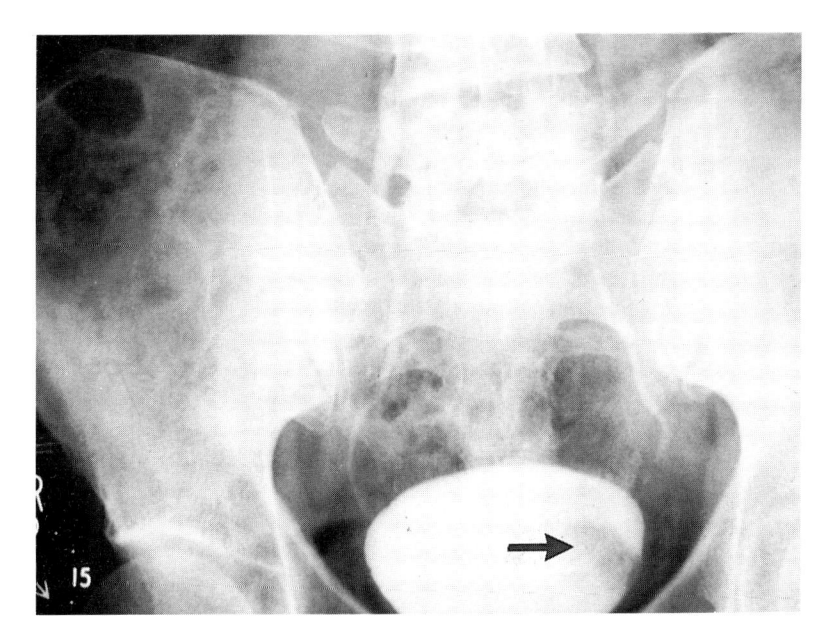

Fig. 17.4 IVU showing a bladder with a filling defect on the patient's left, caused by a bladder carcinoma.

are usually not detected until the patient is unwell from generalized metastatic disease.

Treatment and follow-up

No plan of treatment can be made until the carcinoma has been graded and staged. However, at the diagnostic cystoscopy all tumours that are clinically T2 or less (unless very large) should be removed by transurethral resection.

Non-invasive tumours

After clearance of the original tumour (which may take more than one operation for large or multiple tumours), the patient is followed up by regular cystoscopy. At first the interval should be 3 months, but as the pattern of local recurrence becomes apparent the interval can be varied. Nearly all non-invasive tumours can be managed by cystoscopic surgery. Additional local treatment will help in cases with frequent and numerous recurrences. Cystectomy is required rarely for uncontrolled local disease.

Adjuvant treatment for non-invasive disease: Many modalities are available and the response rates are encouragingly high. Which technique will work for which patient is unpredictable, so the clinician must be prepared to change patient's therapy from one to another.

Intravesical chemotherapy, with thiotepa, epodyl, mitomycin or adriamycin, is usually tried first. Immunotherapy with intravesical BCG and prolonged compression with an intravesical balloon are occasionally useful.

Disease progression: About 25 per cent of cases that are non-invasive at presentation will progress in grade, stage or both. Constant vigilance is essential. Progress usually occurs in bladders showing continuous high rates of recurrence and in tumours that were moderately or poorly differentiated at presentation. However, even well-differentiated and non-invasive tumours can metastasize. If progression occurs the patient is treated as having invasive disease (see below).

Invasive tumours

Invasive tumours require radical treatment. The majority of patients do not have demonstrable metastases at presentation and treatment is aimed at a cure. However, even in cases with suspected or proven metastases, local treatment may be justified because of severe pelvic symptoms. Death from uncontrolled pelvic disease is very unpleasant.

Cases with superficial muscle invasion (T2) are usually treated by radical radiotherapy (65 grey in 6½ weeks). More deeply invasive cancers require preoperative radiotherapy (20-50 gray) and radical cystectomy provided the patient is fit enough. Some urologists use radical radiotherapy for all cases and reserve cystectomy for those who do not respond.

Transitional cell carcinoma of the kidney and ureter

Tumours in these sites should be staged and graded as well as their inaccessible position allows. Small, non-invasive tumours of the renal pelvis can be resected, but the majority require nephroureterectomy. To avoid recurrence in the non-functional ureter, it should be removed en-bloc, including a cuff of bladder. Small, non-invasive ureteric tumours are treated by resection and ureteric anastomosis; more aggressive ones by nephroureterectomy. All patients must undergo regular cystoscopy to look for recurrent carcinoma in the bladder.

Carcinoma of the urethra

The proximal five-sixths of the urethra is lined with urothelium and may be involved in urothelial carcinoma. Primary squamous carcinoma of the male urethra is common in Africa and America, usually as a complication of long-standing stricture. In the United Kingdom it is rare, and the majority arise *de novo* in women. It is treated by radical excision.

Prognosis

The prognosis is closely related to local grade, and stage T1 tumours have a 5-year survival of 70-95 per cent according to grade. Once muscle invasion has occurred mortality increases rapidly: 50-60 per cent of T2 cases and 15-35 per cent of T3 cases survive 5 years. Once the disease has spread to other pelvic organs, fewer than 5 per cent of patients survive 5 years.

Other bladder tumours

Squamous carcinoma

Squamous carcinoma of the bladder usually follows chronic irritation such as occurs in bilharzia or with bladder stones. It is common, therefore, in countries where these conditions are endemic and rare elsewhere. Nearly all are invasive at presentation. They are treated by radical cystectomy with or without preoperative radiotherapy.

Adenocarcinoma

Primary adenocarcinoma of the bladder is very rare. It occurs in the urachal remanent and presents with bladder symptoms. Treatment is by removal of the urachus, the umbilicus and dome of the bladder en-bloc. Adenocarcinoma of the neighbouring large bowel may invade the bladder.

Cancer of the prostate

Carcinoma of the prostate is the third commonest cancer in males. It is quite unlike bladder cancer in its natural history - it metastasises early so that remote symptoms occur relatively early in the disease.

There are no known direct aetiological factors. However, it becomes commoner with increasing age, and by the ninth decade foci of carcinoma can be found in nearly all prostates.

Pathology

The overwhelming majority of prostate cancers are adenocarcinomas. Sarcomas occur rarely in the prostate. The prostatic ducts are lined with transitional epithelium and can, therefore, be involved in urothelial carcinoma.

The common prostatic cancer is a columnar adenocarcinoma with distortion of normal architecture. Several schemes for assessing differentiation exist and correlate reasonably well with prognosis.

Staging

Although the criteria for staging are well recognized, in practice staging is difficult and therefore inaccurate. The staging devised by the UICC is shown in Figure 17.5.

186 *Cancer of the genitourinary tract*

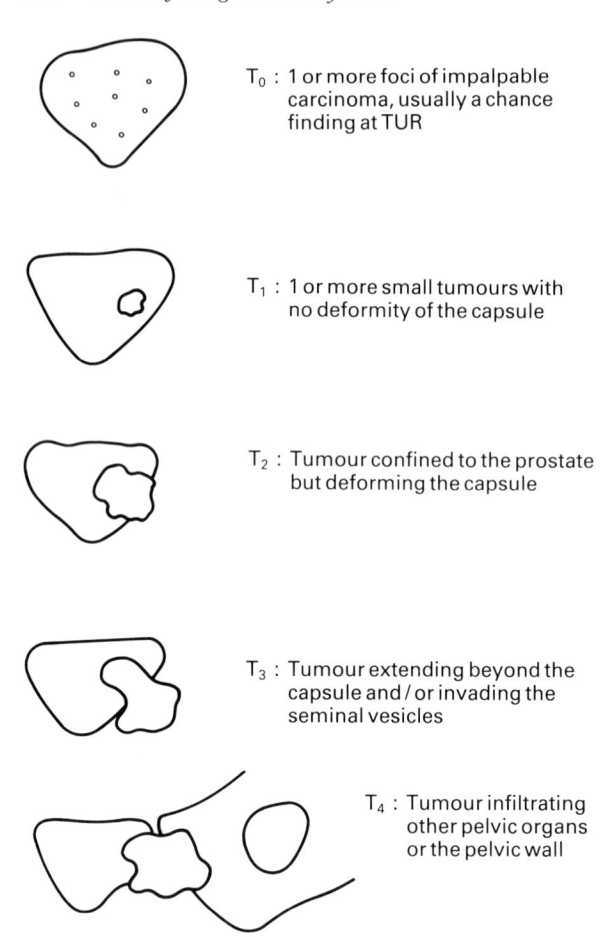

T_0 : 1 or more foci of impalpable carcinoma, usually a chance finding at TUR

T_1 : 1 or more small tumours with no deformity of the capsule

T_2 : Tumour confined to the prostate but deforming the capsule

T_3 : Tumour extending beyond the capsule and / or invading the seminal vesicles

T_4 : Tumour infiltrating other pelvic organs or the pelvic wall

Fig. 17.5 Staging of prostate carcinoma: TNM system.

Presentation

Local disease

Ninety per cent of carcinomas arise in the peripheral zone of the prostate, and therefore small tumours may not interfere with voiding. As they enlarge they obstruct the outflow from the bladder, causing poor stream, frequency and nocturia. Some cancers, however, may grow quite large without causing urinary obstruction: those extending upwards may invade the trigone, causing bladder irritation; a few extend posteriorly, causing tenesmus or even rectal obstruction. Many men present with bladder outflow obstruction caused by benign prostatic hypertrophy and are incidentally found to have a carcinoma as well. Recently the popularity of regular health checks has identified patients with no symptoms.

Remote disease

Cancer of the prostate metastasises early to pelvic lymph nodes and bone. About 15 per cent of T1 tumours, 30 per cent of T2 tumours and 60 per cent of T3 tumours have lymph node metastases at presentation. Half of those with nodal metastases have bone metastases. Patients may present with bone pain, pathological fractures or even anaemia.

Investigations

Urine

The urine frequently contains microscopic quantities of blood, but other tests are unhelpful. Urine cytology is nearly always negative.

Blood

Disseminated metastases in bone may cause anaemia by marrow replacement. Bilateral ureteric obstruction causes raised urea and creatinine. Acid phosphatase is produced by some prostatic carcinomas, but also by a very wide range of normal cells. It is possible to distinguish the fraction of the total acid phosphatase that is of prostatic origin because it is the only portion not inhibited by tartrate. Prostatic acid phosphatase is raised in 5 per cent of cases without metastases and in about 60 per cent of cases with extensive metastases. Its measurement is, therefore, of no use in diagnosis or staging. It can be used to monitor the response to treatment.

Radiology and other imaging

Conventional radiology has little to offer in diagnosing the primary. Transrectal or transurethral ultrasound allows more precise measurement of primary size than is possible with the finger alone. For metastases the first investigation should be a radio-isotope bone scan which will show metastases 3–6 months before there are radiological abnormalities. If a bone scan is negative, nodal metastases should be looked for by bipedal lymphangiography or computerized axial tomography.

Biopsy

The diagnosis of carcinoma of the prostate must never be made without histological or cytological proof. If the patient presents with symptoms of bladder outflow obstruction requiring prostatic resection, tissue will be available for histology. Otherwise suspected cancers should be biopsied by a transperineal or transrectal route. Needle aspiration by these routes for cytology is a good alternative.

Treatment of localized disease

An obstructing prostate requires transurethral resection. In the presence of an obstructing carcinoma, surgery should be conservative as it is all too easy to make the patient incontinent.

If there are no metastases the disease may be curable. Radical treatment is justified if the patient's age and general condition allow – carcinoma of the prostate may grow slowly in some cases so that such treatment may be contraindicated in the elderly man. In England radical treatment means radiotherapy which, although unpleasant and complicated by side-effects in some cases, leaves the patient with a working bladder. Some centres in America and in Europe favour radical prostatectomy, especially if the primary is 2-3 cm in diameter or less. This operation results in incontinence for 10 per cent and impotence for 100 per cent of patients except in the most skilled hands.

Treatment of generalized disease

There is no cure once metastases have occurred, but in some cases progression may be so slow that the patient dies of other causes before the cancer kills him. Although there are several treatments available for advanced disease, there is still some doubt as to whether they slow the progress of the disease or merely give symptomatic relief.

Hormones

In 1941 Huggins and Hodges reported the dramatic effects of castration or oestrogen administration on metastatic prostate cancer. Hormone manipulation has been popular ever since. Therapeutically, orchidectomy and stilboestrol (1 mg t.d.s) are of equal effectiveness. Stilboestrol causes many side-effects, the most serious of which is fluid retention: this limits its use in patients with a history of cardiovascular disease. Orchidectomy is probably the treatment of choice.

Radiotherapy

Localized, symptomatic bone metastases are treated by low dose radiotherapy. However, as one symptomatic metastasis is often followed by several more, some centres irradiate half the body in low dose – upper or lower half as appropriate. The other half can be irradiated later, if necessary, when the bone marrow has recovered.

Drugs

No cytotoxic chemotherapeutic drugs are of proven benefit. Combinations of drugs have given promising results (especially adriamycin, mitomycin and 5-FU), but at the price of severe toxicity. Aminoglutethamide suppresses the adrenal steroids, producing a 'medical adrenalectomy': about 60 per cent of patients achieve useful palliation of generalized bone pain for up to a year or, occasionally, longer.

Surgery

Even in advanced cases limited local resection may be valuable to remove prostatic obstruction. Hypophysectomy relieves bone pain in 30 per cent of cases.

Prognosis

It is very difficult to give a prognosis for an individual patient as the natural history is so uncertain. Patients with one or two foci of carcinoma, in an otherwise benign gland (T0), and those with small cancers without metastases, have the same life expectancy as age-matched controls. The prognosis becomes progressively poorer with increasing stage and grade: for example, the overall survival of T2 cases is about 50 per cent at 5 years. The age of the patient at presentation is irrelevant.

Cancer of the testis

Cancer of the testis is one of the rarest neoplasms. It is of the highest importance, however, because of the young age of patients and the very high cure rates that are achieved by modern aggressive treatment. The proper management requires the combined care of surgeon, radiotherapist and chemotherapist.

Aetiology

Boys with one or two undescended testes at birth are 30 times more likely to develop cancer of the testis than normal boys. The higher the testis the greater the risk of cancer. In unilateral cryptorchism the normally descended testis is also at risk, though less so than the non-descended one. Successful orchidopexy does not appear to alter the risk. There is also an increased risk of tumour in infertile men with oligozoospermia, even with normally descended testes: testicular biopsies have shown areas of carcinoma *in situ* in men who have subsequently developed tumours.

Pathology

Any cells in the testis can give rise to a neoplasm. By far the commonest arise from spermatogonia and are, therefore, known as germ cell tumours. The pathology can be confusing for the student because of the many sub-types that are described. It is easiest to consider them as 'seminomas' and 'non-seminomatous germ cell tumours', the latter being loosely called 'teratomas'.

Seminomas are commonly smooth lumps on the testis with a cut surface that is grossly uniform. Microscopically they consist of sheets of cells similar to spermatogonia. Peak incidence is in the fourth decade, but it can occur at any age after puberty and there is a further, but smaller, peak of incidence in the sixth decade. They occasionally produce alkaline phosphatase.

Non-seminomatous germ cell tumours have a wide variety of gross appearances within a single example and from case to case. There are cystic and solid areas, and even islands of bone or cartilage. This is reflected in the histology – many different fetal and adult tissues appear and are responsible for the pathological sub-divisions. They occur in younger adults than seminomas, with a peak incidence in the third decade; presentation after 30 years old is rare.

Some tumours contain both seminoma and teratoma and are known as 'combined tumours', but the teratoma may be very small: it is most important to recognize the teratomatous element as such tumours behave as teratomas and must be treated accordingly. Germ cell tumours before puberty are nearly always teratomas and metastasise in up to 40 per cent of cases.

The fetal elements in the tumour produce distinct proteins that can be recognized and quantified in the peripheral blood. In general the metastases produce the same as the primary and they are used as tumour markers to monitor the progress of treatment and the appearance of metastases. Trophoblastic areas produce human chorionic gonadotrophin (HCG) and yolk sac elements produce alpha-feto-protein (AFP). Other elements occasionally produce liver enzymes.

Presentation

The overwhelming majority of patients present with a painless swelling of the testis. The testis is sometimes described as feeling 'heavy' or 'numb'. Occasionally the lump is painful, and about 1 per cent of patients present with frank orchitis.

A few patients present with symptoms from metastases – backache, chest pain or breathlessness – gynaecomastia from the HCG production. The primary tumour may have been neglected by patient or doctor, or may be impalpable. Earlier diagnosis by self-examination should be encouraged.

Management

All patients with a painless lump in the testis must be assumed to have a tumour and be treated accordingly. Other causes of such lumps which do not require orchidectomy are very rare. (It is assumed that clinicians can tell the difference between lumps in the testis and lumps entirely confined to the epididymis!) Patients must be treated urgently.

Preliminary investigations

Apart from investigations required to establish the patient's fitness for surgery, the only essential is to take blood for AFP, HCG and liver enzymes.

Surgery

In all cases of suspected testicular tumour, incision is made in the groin and the cord occluded with a non-crushing clamp. The testis is then delivered into the wound. If it is confirmed that there is a lump in the testis, orchidectomy is performed, ligating and dividing the cord proximal to the clamp so that no malignant cells are released into the circulation. Incising the tumour for inspection or biopsy is dangerous, and frozen section histology is often unhelpful. In a patient who only has one testicle, it may be justified to biopsy the testis, return it to the scrotum and do an orchidectomy a day or so later when the diagnosis is confirmed.

Staging

The commonly used staging system is shown in Fig. 17.6. Accurate staging is essential for proper management. Fortunately, germ cell tumours metastasise in an orderly fashion to the ipsilateral para-aortic lymph nodes, thence to the thoracic and supraclavicular nodes. Generalized metastases occur late. Radiological staging depends on computerized axial tomography and lymphangiography. If tumour markers were raised before orchidectomy and fail to disappear from the circulation, or reappear after orchidectomy, metastases are present and their site must be identified.

Treatment

Seminoma

Radiotherapy and chemotherapy are extremely effective in pure seminoma, and cure has been the rule for many years. It is traditional to irradiate one area beyond that in which metastases have been demonstrated: for example, stage 1 tumours get irradiation of the ipsilateral pelvic and both sides of para-aortic nodes; stage 2 tumours get the same plus mediastinal irradiation.

It has recently been shown that single-agent chemotherapy, especially cisplatinum, is highly effective. This opens the way to a 'watch policy' for stage 1 similar to that already established for teratoma. Present regimes give a 90–95 per cent cure rate.

Teratoma

Teratomas are not as radiosensitive as seminomas, and until the advent of combination chemotherapy in the 1960s they had a poor prognosis. Now, however, chemotherapy is so successful that death from teratoma is uncommon.

Stage 1 disease (confined to the testis) is best managed by orchidectomy alone. Patients who relapse have chemotherapy. More advanced cases are treated with chemotherapy (usually bleomycin, vinblastine and VP16 or cisplatinum). Surgery for metastases is needed for any residual disease after chemotherapy.

Non-germ cell testicular tumours

Because all the testicular and paratesticular tissues can give rise to neoplasms, a

Cancer of the genitourinary tract

Staging of testicular tumours
(Royal Marsden Hospital System)

Stage 1: Tumour confined to the testicle

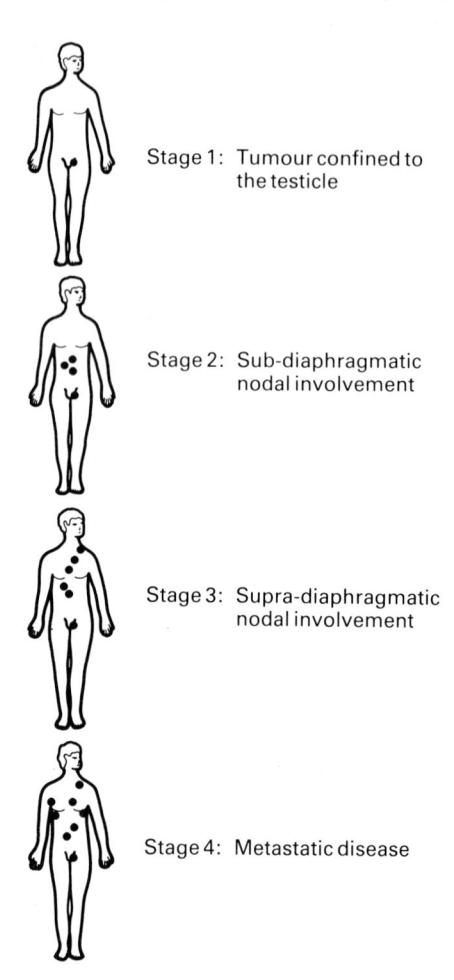

Stage 2: Sub-diaphragmatic nodal involvement

Stage 3: Supra-diaphragmatic nodal involvement

Stage 4: Metastatic disease

Fig. 17.6 Staging of testicular tumours.

wide variety of very rare tumours occur. The supporting cells within the seminiferous tubules are called Sertoli cells. Their precise function is unknown. Their tumours present in adolescence and are commonly benign. They secrete oestrogens, causing gynaecomastia.

The cells between the tubules are called interstitial or Leydig cells. They probably secrete androgens, and their tumours certainly do. In childhood the tumours cause premature sexual development (the Infant Hercules syndrome). They rarely metastasise.

The reticuloendothelial tissue gives rise to lymphomas, either as part of a general disease or in isolation. They occur in old men and may be bilateral. The testis is the commonest site for solid lesions in childhood acute leukaemias, outside the reticuloendothelial system.

Tumours may arise outside the testis and are known as paratesticular. The commonest of a very rare group is the adenomadoid tumour of the epididymis which is benign.

Cancer of the penis

Aetiology

Traditionally cancer of the penis is a disease of 'dirty old men'. This caricature is incorrect nowadays. It is thought to arise in the prepuce and is, therefore, virtually unknown in people who were fully circumcised at birth. It is very rare in England, accounting for about 100 deaths per year. In Uganda, Muslim areas of India and parts of China it is more common. It seems that circumcision at any time beyond the neonatal period is an incomplete protection.

Presentation

Presentation is nearly always as an ulcerating, partly necrotic and infected mass on the distal penis. Occasionally the more observant male will notice a patch of carcinoma *in situ* on the glans or prepuce. In ulcerating cases the inguinal nodes are virtually always enlarged, most commonly from the secondary infection. Treatment of the primary lesion will lead to shrinkage of the nodes, unless they contain metastases. Doubtful nodes should be aspirated for cytology.

Treatment

Penile carcinoma is superficial and squamous cell in origin. All ulcerating lesions should be treated with local cleaning and antibiotics to clear the worst of the infection. All cases should be circumcised and biopsied. For *in situ* lesions and frank carcinoma not invading the corpora cavernosa, partial or total phallectomy is necessary. Nodal involvement requires lymphadenectomy or radiotherapy. The prognosis, especially for early disease, is good.

Further reading

Surgical

Blandy, J.P. (1978). *Operative Urology*. Blackwell Scientific Publications, Oxford.
Chisholm, G.D. and Williams, D.I. (1982). *Scientific Foundations of Urology* (2nd Edn). Heinemann Medical Books, London.
McDougal, W.S. (1986). *Rob and Smith's Operative Surgery – Urology* (4th Edn). Butterworths, London.
Murphy, L.J.T. (1972). *The History of Urology*. Charles C. Thomas, Springfield.
Walsh, P.C., Gittes, R.F. Perlmutter, A.D. and Stamey, T.A. (1986). *Campbell's Urology* (5th Edn. 3 Vols). W.B. Saunders, Philadelphia.
Whitfield, H.N. and Hendry, W.F. (1985). *Textbook of Genitourinary Surgery* (2 Vols). Churchill Livingstone, Edinburgh.
Wickham, J.E.A. (1979). *Urinary Calculous Disease*. Churchill Livingstone, Edinburgh.
Wickham, J.E.A. (1984). *Intra-renal Surgery*. Churchill Livingstone, Edinburgh.

Medical

Catto, G.R.D. and Smith, J.A.R. (1981). *Clinical Aspects of Renal Physiology*. Baillière Tindall, London.
Earle, D.P. (1982). *Manual of Clinical Nephrology*. W.B. Saunders, Boston.
Heptinstall, R.H. (1983). *Pathology of the Kidney*. Little Brown, Boston.
Marsh, F.P. (Ed.) (1985). *Postgraduate Nephrology*. Heinemann Medical Books, London.
Strauss, M.B. and Welt, L.G. (Ed.) (1971). *Diseases of the Kidney* (2nd Edn). Little Brown, Boston.

Chapter 2 Imaging in urology

Sherwood, T. (1978). *Uroradiology*. Blackwell Scientific Publications, Oxford.
O'Reilly, P.H., Shields, R.A. and Testa, J.J. (1979). *Nuclear Medicine in Urology and Nephrology*. Butterworths, London.

Resnick, M.I. and Sanders, R.C. (1984). *Ultrasound in Urology* (2nd Edn). Williams and Wilkins, Baltimore.

Chapter 3 Acute renal failure

Anderson, R.J. and Schrier, R.W. (1980). Clinical spectrum of oliguric and non-oliguric acute renal failure. In *Contemporary Issues in Nephrology* (Vol. 6, pp. 1-16), Ed. B.M. Brenner and J.H. Stein. Churchill Livingstone, Edinburgh.

Chapman, A. (Ed.) (1980). *Acute Renal Failure.* Churchill Livingstone, Edinburgh.

Espinel, C.H. and Gregory, A.W. (1980). Differential diagnosis of acute renal failure. *Clin. Nephrol.* **13**, 73.

Kennedy, A.C., Burton, J.A., Luke, R.G. *et al.* (1973). Factors affecting the prognosis in acute renal failure. *Quart. J. Med.* **42**, 73-86.

Oken, D.E. (1976). Local mechanisms in the pathogenesis of acute renal failure. *Kidney Int.* **10**, 594-599.

Chapter 4 Chronic renal failure

Brenner, B.M., Mayer, T.W. and Hostetter, T.H. (1982). Dietary protein intake and the progressive nature of kidney disease. *New Engl. J. Med.* **307**, 652-659.

Bricker, N.S. (1982). Sodium homeostasis in chronic renal disease. *Kidney Int.* **21**, 886-897.

Curtis, J.R. and Williams, G.B. (1975). *Clinical Management of Chronic Renal Failure.* Blackwell Scientific Publications, Oxford.

Wills, M.R. (1971). *Biochemical Consequences of Chronic Renal Failure.* Harvey Miller and Medcalf, Aylesbury.

Chapter 5 Dialysis

Amir, P., Khanna, R., Leibel, B. *et al.* (1982). Continuous ambulatory peritoneal dialysis in diabetes with end stage renal disease. *New Engl. J. Med.* **306**, 625-630.

Dodd, N.J., O'Donovan, R.M., Bennett-Jones, D.N. *et al.* (1983). Arterio-venous haemofiltration: a recent advance in the management of renal failure. *Brit. Med. J.* **287**, 1008-1010.

Kanis, J.A., Candy, T., Earnshaw, M. *et al.* (1979). Treatment of renal bone disease with 1α-hydroxylated derivatives of vitamin D_3. *Quart. J. Med.* **48**, 289-322.

Nolph, K.D. (1981). Continuous ambulatory peritoneal dialysis. *Nephrology* **1**, 1.

Chapter 6 Transplantation

McGeown, M. (1985). Clinical aspects of transplantation. In *Postgraduate Nephrology* (Ch. 23), Ed. F.P. Marsh. William Heinemann Medical Books, London.

Morris, P.J. (Ed.) (1984). *Kidney Transplantation: Principles and Practice* (2nd Edn). Grune and Stratton, New York.

Vollmer, W.M., Wahl, P.W. and Blagg, C.R. (1983). Survival with dialysis and transplantation in patients with end stage renal disease. *New Engl. J. Med.* **308**, 1553–1558.

Chapter 7 Proteinuria

Cameron, J.S. (1977). Clinicopathological correlates in glomerulonephritis: problems and limitations. *Clin. Nephrol.* **4**, 1–7.

Cameron, J.S. (1982). Glomerulonephritis: current problems and understanding. *J. Lab. Clin. Med.* **99**, 755–787.

Darmady, E.M. and McIver, A.G. (1970). *Renal Pathology*. Butterworths, London.

Chapter 8 Hypertension

Atkinson, A.B., Brown, J.J., Cumming, A.M.M. *et al.* (1982). Captopril in renovascular hypertension: long term use in predicting surgical outcome. *Brit. Med. J.* **1**, 689–693.

Barger, A.C. (1979). Experimental renovascular hypertension. *Hypertension* **1**, 447–455.

Brown, J.J., Lever, A.F., Robertson, J.I.S. and Schalekamp, M.A. (1976). Pathogenesis of essential hypertension. *Lancet* **i**, 1217–1219.

Daggett, P. (1981). *Clinical Endocrinology*. Edward Arnold, London.

Davies, J.O. (1977). The pathogenesis of chronic renovascular hypertension. *Circ. Res.* **40**, 439–444.

Chapter 9 Infections of the urinary tract

Asscher, A.W. (1980). *The Challenge of Urinary Tract Infections*. Academic Press, London.

Gow, J.G. (1981). The management of genitourinary tuberculosis. In *Recent Advances in Urology/Andrology* (3rd Edn, Ch. 7), Ed. W.F. Hendry. Churchill Livingstone, Edinburgh.

Kisner, C.D. (1981). Therapy for tropical urological diseases. In *Recent Advances in Urology/Andrology* (3rd Edn, Ch. 8), Ed. W.F. Hendry. Churchill Livingstone, Edinburgh.

Stamey, T.A. (1980). *Pathogenesis and Treatment of Urinary Tract Infections*. Williams and Wilkins, Baltimore.

Chapter 10 Obstruction

Daggett, P. (1981). *Clinical Endocrinology*. Edward Arnold, London.

O'Reilly, P.H. (1986). *Obstructive Uropathy*. Springer Verlag, Berlin.

Chapter 11 Disorders of bladder function

Blandy, J.P. (1971). *Transurethral Resection*. Pitman, London.
Lloyd-Davies, R.W., Gow, J.G. and Davies, D.R. (1983). *A Colour Atlas of Urology*. Wolfe, London.
Mundy, A.R., Stephenson, T.P. and Wein, A.J.R. (1984). *Urodynamics - Principles, Practice and Application*. Churchill Livingstone, Edinburgh.

Chapter 12 Congenital abnormalities

Kelalis, P.P., King, L.R. and Belman, A.B. (1985). *Clinical Pediatric Urology* (2nd Edn., 2 Vols). W.B. Saunders, Philadelphia.
Stephens, F.D. (1983). *Congenital Malformations of the Urinary Tract*. Praeger, New York.
Williams, D.I. and Johnston, J.H. (1982). *Paediatric Urology* (2nd Edn). Butterworths, London.

Chapter 13 Infertility and impotence

Bennett, A.H. (1982). *Management of Male Impotence*. Williams and Wilkins, Baltimore.
Daggett, P. (1981). *Clinical Endocrinology*. Edward Arnold, London.
Findlay, A.L.R. (1984). *Reproduction and the Fetus*. Edward Arnold, London.
Mann, T. and Lutwak-Mann, C. (1981). *Male Reproductive Function and Semen*. Springer Verlag, Berlin.
Steele, S.J. (1985) *Gynaecology, Obstetrics and the Neonate*. Edward Arnold, London.

Chapter 14 Tubular defects

Berl, T., Anderson, R.J., McDonald, K.M. *et al.* (1976). Clinical disorders of water metabolism, *Kidney Int.* **10**, 117-132.
Daggett, P. (1981). *Clinical Endocrinology* (Chap. 6). Edward Arnold, London.
Segal, S. (1976). Disorders of renal amino acid transport, *New Eng. J. Med.* **294**, 1004.
Stanbury, J.B., Wyngaarden, J.B., Fredricksen, D.S., Goldstein, J.L. and Brown, M.S. (Eds.) (1982). *The Metabolic Basis of Inherited Disease* (5th Edn). McGraw-Hill, New York.
Wrong, O.M. and Feest, T.G. (1982). Renal tubular acidosis. In *Recent Advances in Renal Medicine* (pp. 243-271), Eds. N.F. Jones and D.K. Peters. Churchill Livingstone, Edinburgh.

Chapter 15 Renal disease in general medicine

Cameron, J.S. and Simmonds, H.A. (1981). Uric acid, gout and the kidney, *J. Clin. Path.* **34**, 1245-1254.
Cannon, P.J. (1978). Medical management of renal scleroderma, *New Engl. J. Med.* **299**, 886-887.

Fanci, A.S., Haynes, B.F. and Katz, P. (1978). The spectrum of vasculitis: clinical, pathologic, immunologic and therapeutic considerations, *Ann. Int. Med.* **89**, 660-665.

Mauer, S.M., Steffes, M.W. and Brown, D.M. (1981). The kidney in diabetes, *Amer. J. Medicine* **70**, 603-612.

Triger, D.R. and Joekes, A.M. (1973). Renal amyloidosis - a fourteen year follow up, *Quart. J. Med.* **42**, 15-40.

Chapter 16 Pharmacology

Bennett, W., Aronoff, G., Morrison, G. *et al.* (1983). Drug prescribing in renal failure: dosing guidelines for adults, *Amer. J. Kidney Dis.* **3**, 155-193.

Marsh, F.P. (1982). Drugs and the kidney. In *Oxford Textbook of Medicine* (Vol. 18, pp. 107-110), Eds. J.G.G. Ledingham, D.A. Warrell and D.J. Weatherall. Oxford University Press, London.

Chapter 17 Cancer of the genitourinary tract

Peckham, M. (1981). *The Management of Testicular Tumours.* Edward Arnold, London.

Skinner, D.G. and De Kernion, J.B. (1978). *Genitourinary Cancer.* W.B. Saunders, Philadelphia.

Zinnge, E. and Wallace, D.M.A. (1985). *Bladder Cancer.* Springer Verlag, Berlin.

Index

Index

Abnormalities *see* Congenital defects
Abscesses
  perinephric 91
  renal 89-90
Acetazolamide, bicarbonate wasting 157
Acidosis 36-7
  dialysis 41
  renal tubular 153-5
Acyclovir 55
Addison's disease 142
Adrenal cortex, Conn's syndrome 77
Albumin, selective proteinuria 57
Alcoholism
  and impotence 142, 143, 145
  nephrotic syndrome 68
Aldosterone, Conn's syndrome 77
Alpha-adrenergic blocking agents 80
Amikacin, chronic prostatitis 87
Aminoaciduria 157
Aminoglutethamide, 'medical adrenalectomy' 189
Aminoglycosides
  nephrotoxicity 22, 56, 170
  in peritoneal dialysis 46
  in pyelonephritis 90-91
  in renal failure 30, 168
Ammonium chloride, in hydrogen ion secretion 8-9
Amphotericin B
  Aspergillus infection 55
  nephrotoxicity 170
  tubular damage 22, 157, 170
Amyloid deposition 162-3
  chronic renal failure 32

kidney shape 24
  and renal carcinoma 175
Amyloid fibrils, electron microscopy 5, 163
Anaemia
  and prostate cancer 187
  and renal failure 27, 38, 78
Angina, calcium antagonists 81
Angiography 25
Angiotensin II
  and captopril 81
  cortical vasoconstriction 21
  in pregnancy 165
Angiotensin/renin stimulation 76
  in renal ischaemia 21
Anticholinergic drugs, in incontinence 116, 118
Antiglomerular basement membrane disease 63, 64
Antilymphocyte globulin, in transplantation 51
Aorta, coarctation 77
Aortic dissection and renal vessels 20
Arteriogram, abscesses 89
Arteriovenous fistula 42-3
Artificial insemination 139
Ascites and oedema 2, 4
Aspergillus, post-transplantation 55
Aspirin, in vasculitis 160
Assessment 1-9
  glomerular filtration rate 7
  history 1-3
  physical examination 3-4
  renal blood flow 7-8
  tubular function 8-9

Index

Assessment *continued*
  urine analysis, macroscopic 4-5
    microscopic 5-7
Atenolol
  in diabetes 159
  in hypertension 80
Azathioprine
  glomerulonephritis 67
  transplantation 51
  and vasculitis 160

Bacterial endocarditis 20
  and embolic renal disease 3
Bacterial infections 82-94
Bacteriuria, symptomless 84-5
Basement membrane antibody specificity 61-3
Benedict's solution, contraindications 4
Beta-adrenergic blocking drugs 79-80
Bethanechol, detrusor function 113
Bladder
  adenocarcinoma 185
  congenital defects 130
  decompensation 110
  denervation 119
  detrusor muscle 106-108
  distension, Helmstein's 118
  diverticula 109
  enlargement, painless 103
  examination *see* Imaging techniques
  in situ carcinoma 181-5
  incontinence *see* Incontinence
  inflammation 2
  intravesical pressure 17
  Marshall-Marchetti-Krantz repair 120
  neuropathic lesions 114-17
  normal function 106-108
  obstruction 102-103, 108-114
  retraining of function 119
  sphincter incompetence 119-20
  squamous carcinoma 185
  trabeculation 109, 114
  transitional cell carcinoma 178-85
  tuberculous lesions 92
  tumours 2, 102-103
  urethral repositioning 120
  urinary diversion 120-22
  urothelial carcinoma 178-85

  voiding 108
  see also specific disorders
Bladder neck dyssynergia 114
  obstruction 103
Bleomycin 191
Blood transfusion
  indications 27
  mismatched 21
  pretransplant 51-2
Blood urea 7-8, 104
  chronic renal failure 34-5
Blood vessels *see* specific names and regions
Blood viscosity 72
Bonano catheter 110
Bone
  osteomalacia, osteosclerosis 38
  pain, prostate carcinoma 187, 189
  parathyroid hormone 37-8
  pathology, and dialysis 37
  periosteal erosions 33, 37-8
Bowel, adenocarcinoma 185
Brain, lesions 116

Caecocystoplasty 94
Calcium homeostasis 157
  in bone disease/renal failure 37-8
  and sodium bicarbonate 37
  see also Phosphate: Vitamin D
Calcium oxalate, stones 105
Calyces, strictures 99
Candida, post-transplant 55
Cannulae, in dialysis 42-3
CAPD *see* Dialysis
Captopril
  converting enzyme inhibitor 78, 81
  nephrotic syndrome 81
Carbachol, detrusor function 113
Carcinogens 179
Cardiac
  failure, diuretics in 26
  function, and hypertension 78
  surgery, acute renal failure 28-9
  tamponade 3
Catecholamines in pregnancy 165
Catheters
  peritoneal dialysis 45-6
  in spinal cord transection 115
  suprapubic 110
  see also Incontinence

Cephalosporins
  peritoneal dialysis 46
  tubular damage 22, 170
Children
  bacteriuria, symptomless 84-5
  bladder neck obstruction 103
  enuresis 117-18
  membrane-proliferative glomerulonephritis 67
  undescended testes 132-4
  vesicoureteric reflux 127-30
  see also Congenital defects
Chlamydia, in prostatitis 86, 87
Chlorthalidone 79
Chordee, and hypospadias 131
Chronic renal failure see Renal failure
Cimetidine, and impotence 143
Circumcision, contraindications, hypospadias 131
Cisplatin
  nephrotoxicity 170
  in testicular cancer 191
Clavicle and humerus, osteodystrophy 33
Clear cell tumour 173
Clearance 7
  see also Creatinine
Clostridium difficile, post-transplant 55
CNS disturbance 27
Coarctation, aorta 77
Colic, ureteric 2
  pethidine in 101
Colon conduit 120-21
Complement cascade 62
Computed tomography 13-14
  kidney size and obstruction 96
Conduits
  continent 122
  ileal 120
  Kock technique 122
  ureterosigmoid 121
  urinary diversion 120-22
Congenital defects 104, 123-35
  of bladder 130
  and impotence 141
  of kidney 123-24
  renal pelvic and ureteric anomalies 124-30
  testes 132-5
  urethra 131, 133
  see also Tubular defects

Conn's syndrome 77
Contrast medium
  in IVU 11, 23
  nephrotoxicity 170
Corneal calcification 4
Coronary artery disease 70, 78
  percutaneous transluminal dilatation 37
  and renal atheroma 75
Cortex
  necrosis 21
    pre-eclampsia 166
  vasoconstriction 21
Cotrimoxazole, in non-specific urethritis 55
  in prostatitis 87
Creatinine clearance
  chronic renal failure 32, 35
  and hypertension 78
  and plasma creatinine 7
Crede manoeuvre 115, 116
Cryptorchism 132-4
CT see Computed Tomography
Cushing's syndrome 142
Cyclophosphamide
  in glomerulonephritis 67
  in vasculitis 160
Cyclosporin A
  nephrotoxicity 170
  transplantation 51, 56
Cystectomy, in carcinoma 184
Cystic disease, chronic renal failure 31
  polycystic disease 24
Cystinosis 153
Cystinuria 152
Cystitis 82-4
  aetiology 82-3
  recurrent, and vesicoureteric reflux 127
  and residual urine 110
  sexual technique 86
  specific problems 85-6
Cystometrograms, video 17
Cystoscopy, tuberculosis 93
Cystourethrograms 12-13
Cytomegalovirus, post-transplant 55
Cytur test 84

DDAVP see Desamino D-8 arginine vasopressin

204 Index

Deafness, and hereditary nephritis 4
Depression, and impotence 149
Desamino D-8 arginine vasopressin 8, 155
Detrusor muscle
  drugs stimulating 113
  failure, in retention 112
  hypertrophy 103
  hypotonia, Parkinsonism 116
  instability 109-10, 118-19
    Parkinsonism 116
  normal function 106-108
Dextrose, in IVU 23
DHCC see Dihydrocholicalciferol 37
Diabetes insipidus 155
Diabetes mellitus 158-9
  chronic renal failure 32
  and impotence 143, 146
Dialysis
  haemodialysis 40-43
  haemofiltration 43-4
  indications 26-7
  peritoneal 44-7
    and CAPD (chronic ambulatory) 40, 46, 159
Diazoxide vasodilation 80
Diet
  chronic renal failure 34
  hyperkalaemia 36
  and sodium retention 35
Diethylene triamine pentacetic acid 8, 15
Digoxin, in renal failure 30, 168
Dihydrocholicalciferol, renal production 37
  see also Vitamin D
Dimercaptosuccinate 15
Dipyridamole
  antiplatelet therapy 67, 160
  in diabetes 159
Distal tubular acidosis 153
Distigmine bromide in detrusor contraction 104, 113
Diuresis
  challenge, acute renal failure 26
  and dialysis 27
  in chronic renal failure 36
  loop diuretics 26
  post-operative 104
DMSA see Dimercaptosuccinate

L-Dopa in Parkinsonism 116
Dormia basket 101
Drug treatment 167-9
  'half-life' 167-8
Drug toxicity 32, 169-70
  agents 22, 170
DTPA see Diethylene triamine penta acetic acid
Duplex kidney 117

Eclampsia 165-6
EDTA see Ethylene-ditetra-acetic acid
Ejaculation 142
  retrograde 111, 137
  and sympathectomy 142
Electrocardiogram, hyperkalaemia 26
Emepromium, incontinence 116
Enuresis 2, 117-18
Eosinophilia, tubular damage 22
Epididymis
  adenomatoid tumour 193
  epididymo-orchiditis 87-8
  painless enlargement 93
Erection
  normal physiology 140-42
  organic/psychogenic factors 142
  impotence 142-9
  priapism 149-50
Ergotamine, retroperitoneal fibrosis 169
Erythropoietin production 38, 52
Escherichia coli
  cystitis 82
  pyelonephritis 88
  in tuberculosis 93
ESR (erythrocyte sedimentation rate), in retroperitoneal fibrosis 102
Ethacrynic acid, diuresis 26
Ethambutol 93-4
Ethylene-ditetra-acetic acid, injection extravasation 7
Exstrophy/epispadias 144
  see also Hypospadias
Extramural lesions 101
Eyes
  corneal calcification 4
  and hypertension 78

Fanconi syndrome 57, 153
Fertility see Impotence: Infertility

Fick principle, renal flow 8
Fluid intake/output
  in chronic renal failure 35-6
  conservation 156
  cystitis 85-6
  management 30
Fluorocytosine 55
Frusemide 26, 36

Gallium isotope scan 88
Gamma camera 14, 24-5
Gentamicin *see* Aminoglycosides
Germ cell tumours, cryptorchism 134
Glomerular filtration rate
  and blood urea 8
  chronic renal failure 32, 34
  clearance measurement 7
Glomerulonephritis 57-70
  acute 63-4
  antibodies, basement membrane 62
  cell proliferation 21
  chronic 31, 64
  clinical presentation 63
  focal 67
  histological classification 58-9
  immunology 61-3
  membranous 66-7, 165
    and sarcoid lesions 165
  nephrotic syndrome 68-70
  post-streptococcal 22
  in pregnancy 166
  proliferative sclerosis 162
    Wegener's granulomatosis 161
  rapidly progressive 64
Glomerulus
  blood vessel occlusion, hypertension 77-8
  histology 58-61
Glucose test 4
Glycine irrigant in prostatectomy 112
Glycosuria, diagnosis 9
Gold, nephrotic syndrome 169
  proteinuria 69
Gonadotrophin releasing hormone 134
Gonococcus neisseria 86
Goodpasture's syndrome 3, 62
Gout 164
Grafts *see* Transplantation
Gubernaculum activity 132-3

Guillain-Barré syndrome 117
Gynaecomastia, HCG, in carcinoma 190, 192

Haematuria 171-3
  in children 173
  glomerulonephritis 63
  in obstruction 96
Haemofiltration 43-4
  and dialysis 27
Haemolytic uraemic syndrome 20, 166
Heart *see* Cardiac
Helmstein's balloon 118
Henoch-Schönlein purpura 162
  and proteinuria 64, 69
Hepato-renal syndrome, tubular dysfunction 21
Herpes simplex, post-transplant 55
Hippuran renogram 14-15
'Horseshoe' kidneys 124
Hydralazine
  in hypertension 28, 80
  lupus-like syndrome 169
Hydrogen ions, normal values 36
  acquired bicarbonate wasting 157
Hydronephrosis, vesicoureteric reflux 127
Hyperacute rejection 51-2
Hypercalcaemia 152, 156
  and myeloma 164
Hypercalciuria 157
  idiopathic 154
Hyperkalaemia
  and diuretics 26, 36
  ECG changes 26
  peritoneal dialysis 44
Hypernephroma 173
Hyperoxaluria 105
Hyperparathyroidism 37-8, 154
Hyperpigmentation 3
Hyperprolactinaemia 142
Hypertension 71-81
  acute renal failure 28-9
  aetiology 72-3
  and cardiac problems 81
  chronic renal disease 31, 37, 76
  end-organ damage 77-8
  essential hypertension 77
  glomerulonephritis 64
  and haematuria 171-2

Hypertension *continued*
  non-renal causes 76-7
  and obstruction 76, 95
  renal artery stenosis 73-6, 78
  renin secreting tumours 76
  renoprival 76
  treatment, alpha-adrenergic
    blockade 80
    beta-adrenergic blockade 79-80
    calcium antagonists 81
    converting enzyme inhibitors 81
    diuretics 79
    vasodilators 80
Hypogonadism 141
Hypokalaemia 156
  Conn's syndrome 77
Hyponatraemia 26
  dilutional 26
  glycine irrigants 112
Hypoparathyroidism 37-8
  pseudohypoparathyroidism 152
Hypophosphataemic rickets 151-2
Hypospadias 131
Hypotension
  postural 80
  tubular dysfunction 21
Hypothyroidism 142
Hypovolaemia, and diuresis 79

Idoxuridine 55
Ileal conduit 120-21
Imaging techniques 10-19
  CT scan 13-14
  cystometrograms 17-18
  cystourethrograms 12-13
  flow rate 16-17
  isotope scans 14-15
  micturating cystourethrogram
    (MCU) 12-13
  nuclear magnetic resonance 18-19
  renography 14-15
  ultrasonography 14
  urethral pressure profile 18
  urograms (IVU) 11-12
  Whitaker test 15-16
  X-rays 10-11
    IVU 11-12
    MCU 12-13
Imipramine, enuresis 118
Immune complex disease 61, 70

Immune response 48-9
  glomerulus involvement 61-63
  and renal failure 27
Immunogammaglobulin/transferrin
  ratio 57-8
Impotence 140-49
  examination 143-7
  following prostatectomy 112
  history 143
  normal function 140-42
  organic/psychogenic 142-3
  treatment 147-9
Incontinence 117-20
  congenital defects 117
  enuresis 117-18
  intermittent 115
  post-prostatectomy 111, 116
  pregnancy and 119-20
  sphincter incompetence 119
  in spinal cord transection 115-16
  'stress' type 116, 119
  urge incontinence 109, 116
Infertility 136-9
  cryptorchism 133
  history 137
  physiology 136-7
  and prostatectomy 111-12
Injection extravasation 8
Inherited defects *see* Congenital defects
Insulin
  -carbohydrate ratio 26
  chronic renal failure 39, 168
  in hyperkalaemia 36
  in peritoneal dialysis 45, 47
'Intact nephron' hypothesis 35
Iodine-hippuran renogram 14-15
Ischaemia, generalized 37
Isoniazid 93-4
  lupus-like syndrome 169
Isotope studies 14-15
  see also Gamma camera: Scintigraphy
IVU *see* Urograms

Kallman's syndrome 141
Kanomycin, tubular damage 22
Kidney
  cancers 173-8
  congenital abnormalities 123-4
  drug damage, susceptibility 169
  enlargement 3-4, 24

and myeloma 164
in obstruction 96-7
'horseshoe' 124
obstruction 98-101
pressure atrophy, tuberculous 92
rejection *see* Transplantation
stones 98-9
calcium oxalate 105
Klebsiella 88
Kussmaul respiration 3

Labetalol in hypertension 29, 80
Left ventricular failure, hypertensive 2, 3, 78
Leriche's syndrome 143
Listeria monocytogenes, post-transplant 55
Liver disease
enlargement 3
hepato-renal syndrome 21
Loop diuretics 26, 36
Lymphocoele, in transplantation 54

Magnesium
loss, post-transplant 157
reabsorption 157
Malaria, nephrotic syndrome 70
'Malignant cystitis' 182
Malignant hypertension, glomeruli 20-21
Mannitol
diuretic challenge 26
in IVU 23
Marshall-Marchetti-Krantz repair 120
Mazindol, in prolapse 120
MCU *see* Micturating cystourethrogram
Medullary sponge kidney 154
Mee's lines 3
Mercaptopurine 48
Mercury
nephrotic syndrome 69
tubular necrosis 69
Metabolic acidosis 36-7
and dialysis 41
Methoxyflurane, tubular damage 22
Methysergide 102
retroperitoneal fibrosis 169
Metronidazole

peritoneal dialysis 46
pseudomembranous colitis 55
Micturating cystourethrogram 12-13
Micturition, normal physiology 106-108
see also Voiding
Milk alkali syndrome 154
Minoxidil, vasodilation 80
Mitral stenosis and renal vessels 20
Multiple myeloma 163-4
chronic renal failure 32
kidney, shape 24
Multiple sclerosis 117
Multistix test 84
haematuria 171
Mycoplasma tuberculosis 91-4
Myeloma *see* Multiple myeloma
Myocardial infarction 70
tubular dysfunction 21
Myoglobinuria, tubular dysfunction 21

NAG (N-Acetylglucosaminidase) 53
Nails, Mee's lines 3
Nalidixic acid, cystitis 86
Neoplasia, bladder squames 6
Nephrocalcinosis 153-4, 157
Nephrograms 24
Nephron, 'intact nephron' hypothesis 35
Nephropathy
analgesic 89
reflux 127-8
Nephrostomy in bladder obstruction 102
Nephrotic syndrome
acute 68-70
pathology 57, 63, 66
and amyloid 163
fat droplets 6
Nephrotoxicity 22, 169-70
Neuropathies 114-16
occult 83
Neurotransmission in normal bladder function 106-108, 140-41
Nifedipine, calcium antagonist 81
Nitrofurantoin, cystitis 86
Nocardia asteroides, post-transplant 55
Noradrenaline, in essential hypertension 77
Nuclear magnetic resonance 18-19

Obstruction 95-105
  acute retention 109-10
  bladder 102-103, 108-14
  in children 104
  chronic retention 112-13
  hypertension 76
  kidney 98-101
  management 104-105
  prostate enlargement 103-104
    see also Prostate
  signs and symptoms 95-7
  of ureter 101-102
Oedema
  glomerulonephritis 63, 66
  presenting feature 2-3
  pulmonary, and dialysis 27
  tubular damage 22
Oligohydramnios 123
Oliguria, physiological/acute dysfunction 22-3
Orchidectomy in prostate carcinoma 188
Osteomalacia in hypophosphataemia 152
Oxalosis 154
Oxybutinine in incontinence 118

Pancreatitis
  polyuria 23
  tubular dysfunction 21
Papaverine, self-injection 149
Papillary necrosis
  causes 156
  diabetic-induced 158
  nephrocalcinosis 154
  renal obstruction 99
  and urothelial cancer 179
Papillary tumours 179
Parathyroid hormone 37, 151
  hyperparathyroidism 37-8, 154
  pseudohypoparathyroidism 152
Parenteral nutrition 43
Parkinson's disease, bladder dysfunction 116
Paroxysmal tachycardia 76
Pelviureteric junction
  artery to lower pole 101
  obstruction 99-100, 124-5
Penicillamine
  in cystinuria 69, 152

nephrotic syndrome 169
Penicillin, glomerulonephritis 64
Penis
  balanitis 148
  carcinoma 193
  circumcision 131
  chordee 146-7, 148
  drug therapy 149
  examination 143-5
  hypospadias 131, 133
  phimosis 148
  priapism 149-50
  prostheses 147-8
  surgery 148-9
Perinephric abscess 91
Peripheral neuropathy 117
  impotence 143
  and myeloma 163
Peritoneal dialysis 44-7
  acute 45
  continuous ambulant 47
Peritonitis, cortical ischaemia 21
Pethidine, in renal colic 101
Peyronie's disease 146
Phaeochromocytoma 76-7
Phalanges, periosteal erosions 33, 37-8
Pharmacology 167-9
Phenacetin
  nephropathy 169
  tubular damage 57
Phenindione, toxicity 170
Phenoxybenzamine, alpha-adrenergic blocker 114
Phenylbutazone, lupus-like syndrome 169
Phenylpropanolamine, in prolapse 120
Phenylketonuria 157
Phenytoin, lupus-like syndrome 169
Phimosis, and impotence 148
Phosphate
  binding, aluminium hydroxide 38
  excretion, renal failure 37
  reabsorption 151-2
Physical examination 3-4
Pitressin, in tubular function 8
Pneumocystis carinii, post-transplant 55
Poisoning, heavy metals 57
Polyarteritis nodosa 20, 161
  glomerulonephritis 64, 68
  and pregnancy 166

Polycystic disease 24, 123-4
Polymixins, tubular damage 22, 170
Polyuria and renal failure 23
Postural hypotension 80
Potassium
  plasma levels 36, 104, 156
    cardiac arrhythmia 26
  see also Hyperkalaemia:
    Hypokalaemia
Prader-Willi syndrome 141
Prazosin, alpha-blocking 80
Prednisolone in transplantation 51
Pre-eclampsia 165-6
Pregnancy
  effect on renal function 165-6
  and polyarteritis nodosa 166
  prolapse, prevention 119-20
Priapism 149-50
Probanthine, in incontinence 116, 118
Probe renograms 24
Prolapse 119-20
Propranolol in hypertension 28, 79-80
Prostaglandin E2, in detrusor function 113
Prostate
  benign prostatic hypertrophy 109-12
  carcinoma 102-103, 185-9
    presentation 186-7
    treatment 188-9
  massage, contraindications 87
  and obstruction 103-104
  'trapped', bladder neck dyssynergia 114
Prostatectomy 111-12
  complications 111
  contraindications 110
  and libido 111-12
  in Parkinsonism 116
  retropubic 111-12
  transurethral resection 111
Prostatitis
  acute 86-7
  chronic bacterial 85, 87
  and sperm count 139
  tuberculous 92
Prostatodynia 87
Prostheses 147-8
Protein
  casts, tubular and collecting duct lumens 6

Tamm-Horsfall protein 6
  tests 5
Proteinuria 57-70
  appearance of urine 2
  common causes 69
  exercise-induced 57
  glomerular damage, immune complex 61
  in glomerulonephritis 63-8, 69
  in nephrotic syndrome 68-9
  non-selective 58
  in obstruction 96
  orthostatic 57
  selective 57-8
Proteus mirabilis
  cystitis 84
  and kidney stones 98
  pyelonephritis 88
Proximal tubular acidosis 153-5
Prune belly syndrome 134
Pseudohypoparathyroidism 152
Pseudomonas 88
Psychiatric illness and prostatodynia 87
Psychosexual therapy 149
PTH see Parathyroid hormone
Pyelograms 24-5
Pyelonephritis 88-9
  chronic renal failure 31
  cystitis 83
Pyonephrosis 90-91
Pyrazinamide 93-4
Pyridoxine in oxalate excretion 105
Pyuria, sterile 93

Radiology see Urograms
Radiotherapy, radical 184
Rejection see Transplantation
Reflux see Vesicoureteric reflux
Renal abscess and carcinoma 89-90
Renal adenocarcinoma 173-8
Renal artery
  and aortic dissection 20
  extra, lower pole 101
  stenosis 73-6, 78
    diagnosis 8
    and dilatation 37
    in transplantation 54
Renal biopsy 25
Renal blood flow 8
  Fick principle 8

Renal calculi *see* Kidney stones
Renal cell carcinoma 173–8
Renal cysts 123–4
Renal failure, acute 20–30
  clinical management 25–9
  daily dialysis 42
  investigations 22–5
  parenchymal damage 5
  pathophysiology 20–22
  recovery phase 30
  spinal cord transection 115–16
Renal failure, chronic 31–9
  aetiology 31–2
  clinical assessment 32–4
  corneal calcification 4
  and diabetes 158–9
  end-stage, Henoch-Schönlein purpura 162
  and hypertension 76
  management 34–9
  prostate enlargement 103–104
  substitution therapy 39
Renal failure, polyuric 23
Renal osteodystrophy 32–3
Renal perfusion index 8
Renal tubular acidosis 153–5
Renal tubules, maximum absorptive capacity (T_m) 9
Renal vein thrombosis 68
Renin-angiotensin system
  hypovolaemia 79
  renal ischaemia 21
  see also Angiotensin
Renograms, in obstruction 97
Respiratory system, examination 3
Retroperitoneum
  fibrosis 102
  neoplastic lesion 101
Rifampicin 93–4
  tubular damage 170

Salicylates, clearance, forced alkaline diuresis 167
Sarcoidosis 154, 165
Scintigraphy
  glomerular filtration rate 8
  kidney function 89
  in obstruction 97–8
  see also Gamma camera: Isotope studies

Scleroderma, vessels 20
Sclerosis, systemic 161–2
Scrotum
  epididymal enlargement 93
  torsion 88
  see also Epididymis
Seminoma 189, 191
Septicaemia, tubular dysfunction 21–2
Serum sickness 62
Sjögren's syndrome and hydrogen ions 157
Smoking, and carcinogens 179
Smooth muscle relaxants, contraindications 101
Sodium balance 155–6
  chronic renal failure 35–6
Sodium bicarbonate, metabolic acidosis 37
Sodium nitroprusside 80
'Space occupying lesion' 175–6
Sperm production 136–9
  agglutinating antibodies 139
  examination 138
  history 137–8
  physiology 136–7
  sperm count 136–7
Sphincter incompetence 119–20
Spinal cord transection, in trauma 115–16
Stenosis *see* Renal artery stenosis
Steroids
  glomerulonephritis 67
  in transplantation 51, 55
  in vasculitis 160
Stilboestrol
  and impotence 143
  in prostate carcinoma 188
Streptococci 88
  glomerulonephritis 63–4
Stress incontinence 116, 119
Strokes, management 116
Substitution therapy 39
Sulphonamides, tubular damage 22, 170
Syphilis 69
Systemic lupus erythematosus 160–61
  and hydrogen ions 157
  and pregnancy 166
Systemic sclerosis 160–62

Index

Tamm-Horsfall protein 6, 57
Teratoma 189, 191
Testes
  bell clapper deformity 134
  cancer 189-93
  congenital abnormalities 132-5
  cryptorchism 132-4
    and carcinoma 189
  non-germ cell tumours 191-3
  torsion 134-5
Tetracycline, nephrotoxicity 170
Thiazides, diuresis 79
Thrombosis, and nephrotic syndrome 68, 70
Thyrotoxicosis 142
Tissue matching 50-51
T_M (tubule absorptive capacity)
  bicarbonate 9
  glucose 9
Tolbutamide, nephrotic syndrome 169
Tomography *see* Computed tomography
Transferrin, selective proteinuria 57
Transitional cell cancer 100, 102, 178-85
  bladder 178-84
  industrial causes 179
  kidney and ureter 184-5
Transplantation 48-56
  blood flow, changes 8
  immunology 48-9
  postoperative management 52-6
    complications 54-6
  rejection damage, clinical signs 5, 49-50
    prevention 50-52
  surgical procedure 52
  survival period 56
Trichomonas, prostatitis 86
Troxidone, nephrotic syndrome 169
Tryptizol enuresis 118
Tuberculosis, genitourinary 91-4
Tubular disorders
  acidosis 153-5
  acquired defects 156-7
  acute necrosis 21
  in graft rejection 50, 54
  specific defects 151-5
Tubules, function 8-9

Ultrafiltration and dialysis 42
  in sodium retention 29
Ultrasound 14
  abscess needling 89
  in renal failure 24, 25
Uraemia, and heart function 3
Urea 7-8, 104
  chronic renal failure 34-5
Ureterograms 13
  antegrade/retrograde 13
  see also Urograms
Ureterosigmoidostomy 121
Ureterovesical junction 103, 110
Ureters
  colic 2, 101
  duplication 126-7
  ectopia 126-7
    crossed 125
  megaureter 130
  obstruction 101-102
  retroperitoneal fibrosis 102
  stones 101
  transitional cell carcinoma 184
  tumours 102
  ureterocoele, upper pole 127, 128
  ureterosigmoidostomy 121
  see also Pelviureteric junction: Vesico-ureteric reflux
Urethra
  carcinoma 184
  congenital abnormalities 131
  diameter 108
  ectopia 124-5
    in girls 126-7
  normal function 106-108
  repositioning 120
  resistance to flow 108
  sphincter, artificial 120
  squamous carcinoma 184
  stricture 113-14
  urothelial carcinoma 184
Urethrograms 12-13
'Urge incontinence' 109
Uric acid
  calculi 164
    see also Kidney stones
  chronic renal failure 35
  and gout 164
Urinary tract
  cancer 178-85

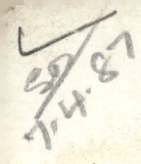

Urinary tract *continued*
  infections 82–94, 182
Urine
  acidification 9
  amino acids 157
  analysis 96, 171
    macroscopic 4–5
    microscopic 5–6
  bacterial examination, cystitis 84
  bacteriuria, symptomless 85
  calciuria 157
  crystals and deposits 6
  dilution test, contraindications 8
  discoloration 2
  diversion 120–22
  electrophoresis 9
  haematuria *see* Haematuria
  haemoglobin, free 5
  microscopy 5–6, 23
  osmolality, and tubular function 8
  parameters, in acute renal failure 23
  passage, disorders in 1–2
    post-emptying of bladder 1
  polyuria 23
  pyuria, sterile 93
  red cells 5, 171
  retention, acute 103–104, 109–110
    chronic 112–13
    see also Obstruction
  sodium concentration 23
  tubular epithelial cells 5
Urodynamics
  cystometrograms 17–18
  flow rate 16–17
Urograms
  intravenous (IVU) 11–12, 24–5
    chronic nephritis 89
    contraindications 110
    in cystitis, certain groups 85
    and fluid deprivation 163
    in obstruction 96–7
    reaction, prophylaxis 11
  micturating
    cystourethrogram 12–13
  ureterograms 13
Urothelium, cancer 178–85

Vancomycin 55
Varicocoele 138
Vasculitis 159–60
Vasoactive intestinal peptide
  nerve endings 143
  vascular neurotransmitter 141
Vasopressin (DDAVP) 155
Vesicoureteric reflux 88–9, 127–30
  lower pole ureter 126
  and PUJ obstruction 124
  and stenosis 130
Videocystometry 17, 110, 114
Vinblastine 191
Vitamin D
  -dependent rickets 152
  disordered metabolism 37–8
  increased sensitivity and serum
    calcium 165
  1α vitamin D 152
  in renal failure 168
  in tubular disorders 152–3
Voiding
  MCU 12–13
  normal 106–108
  reflex, Crede 115–16
  trial of, Bonano catheter 110
VP 16 19

Wegener's granulomatosis 3, 161
Whitaker test 15–16
Wilson's disease 57

Young's syndrome 138

Ziel–Nielson technique 93